THE STORY OF CANCER
Volume 3

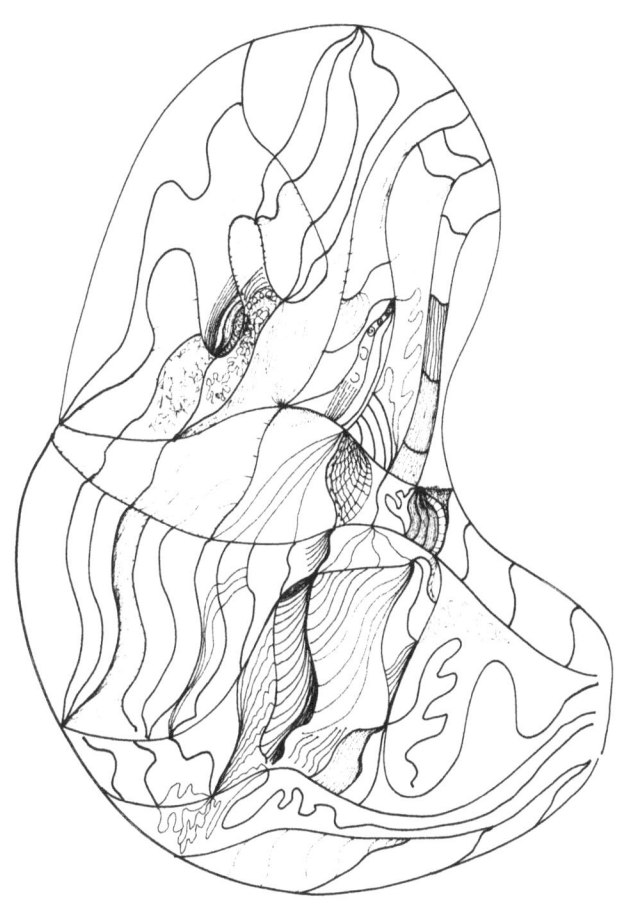

Camilia MacPherson, Ph.D., D.Th.
2016

INTRODUCTION

This is the Story of Cancer told using Automatic Drawings and Surreal Art. It is part of a continuous document written in 7 volumes.

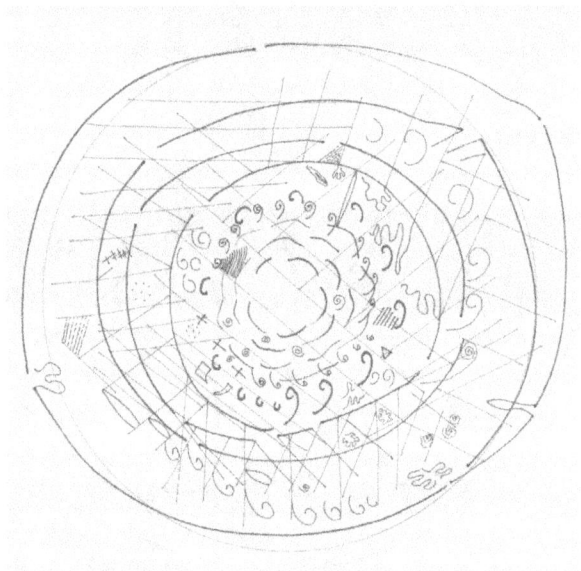

ISBN-13: 978-1530543922
ISBN-10: 1530543924
Email: tamaracpublishers@icloud.com

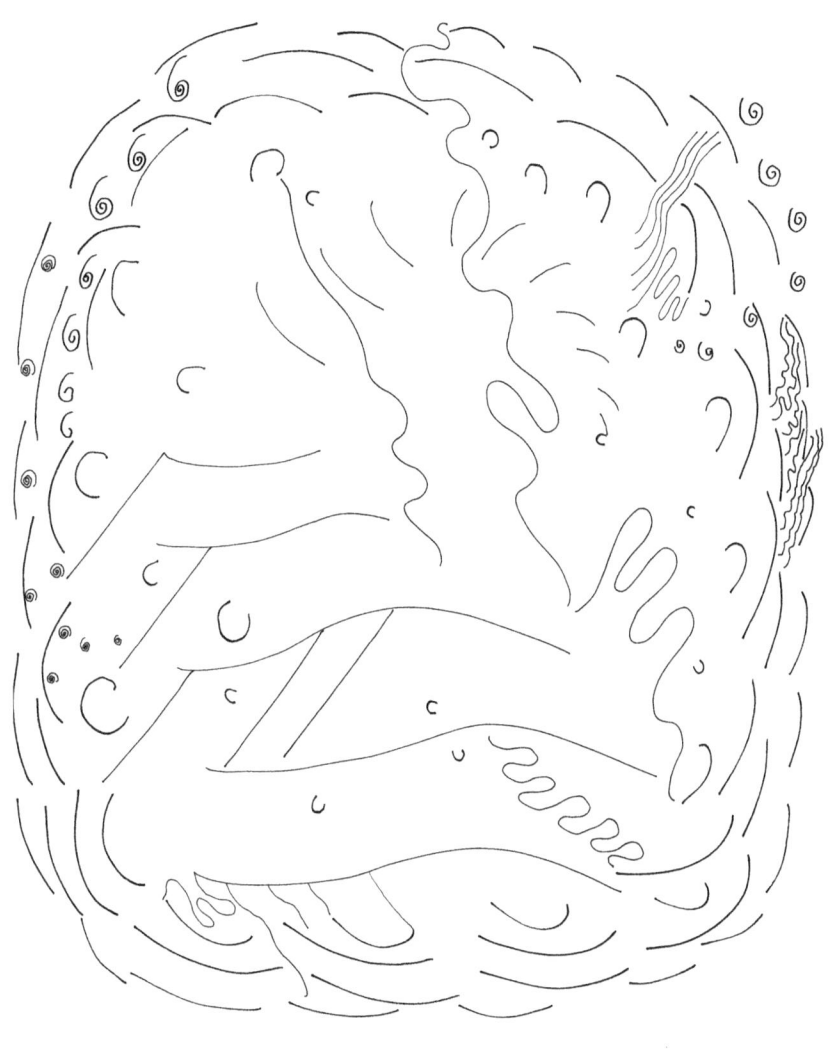

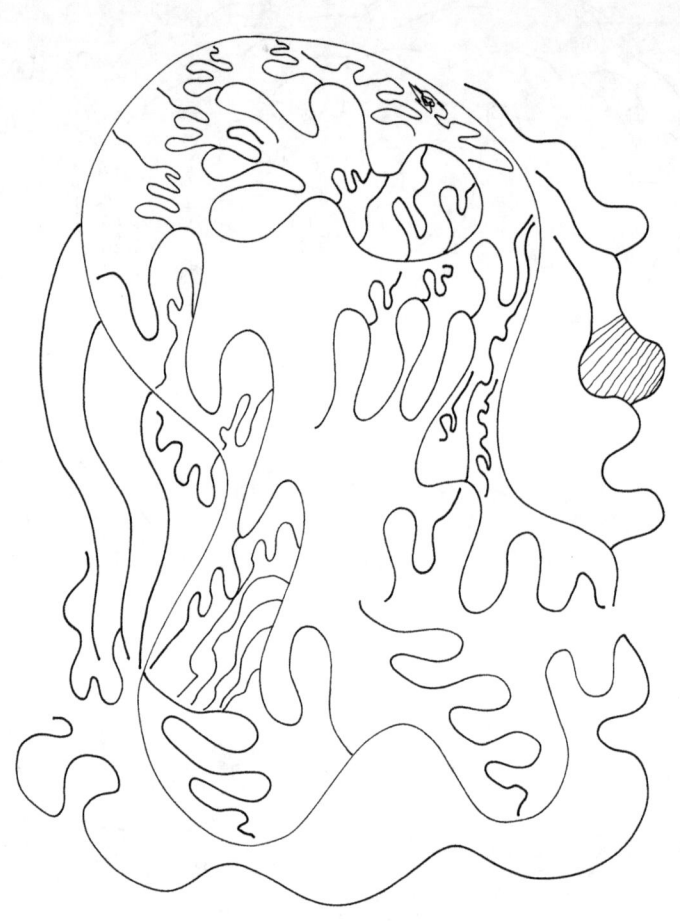

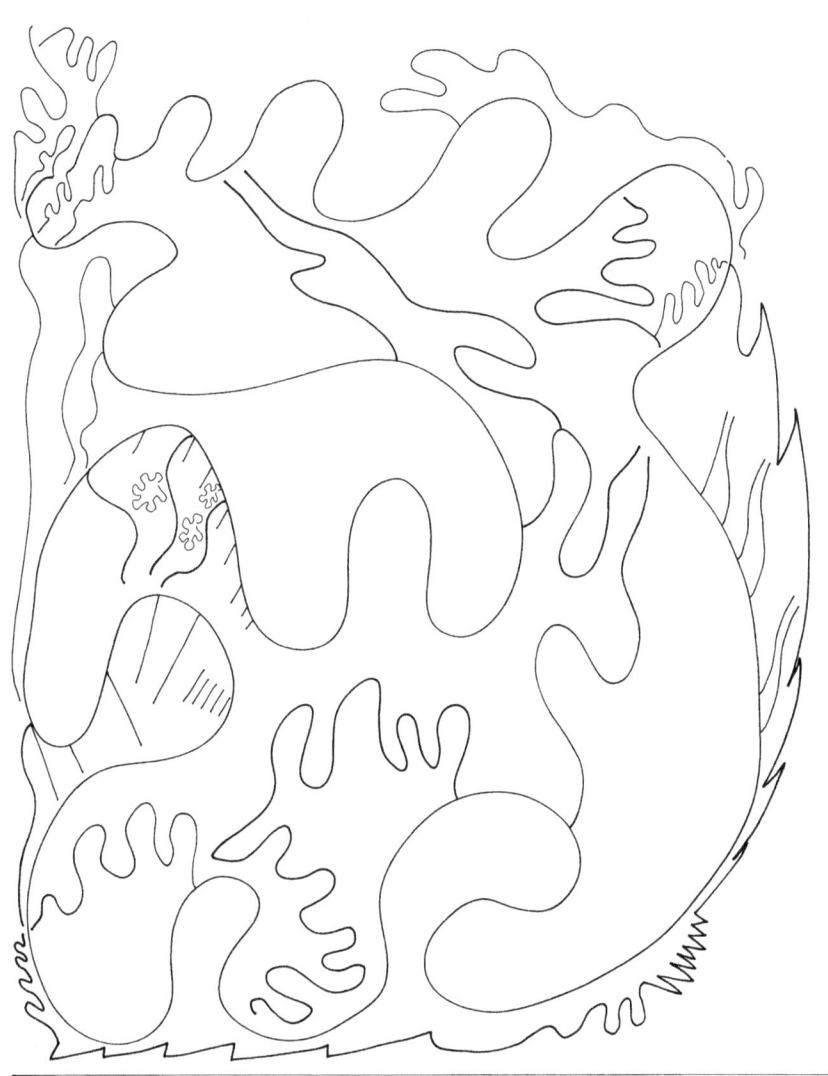

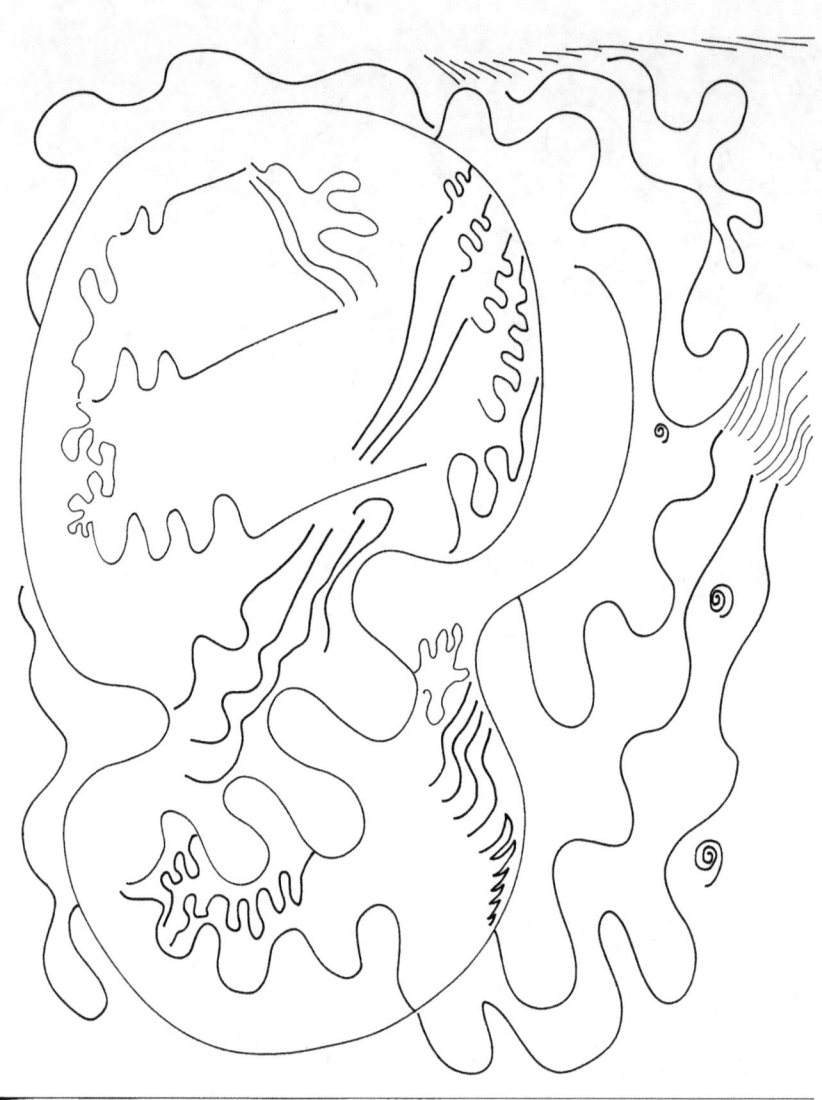

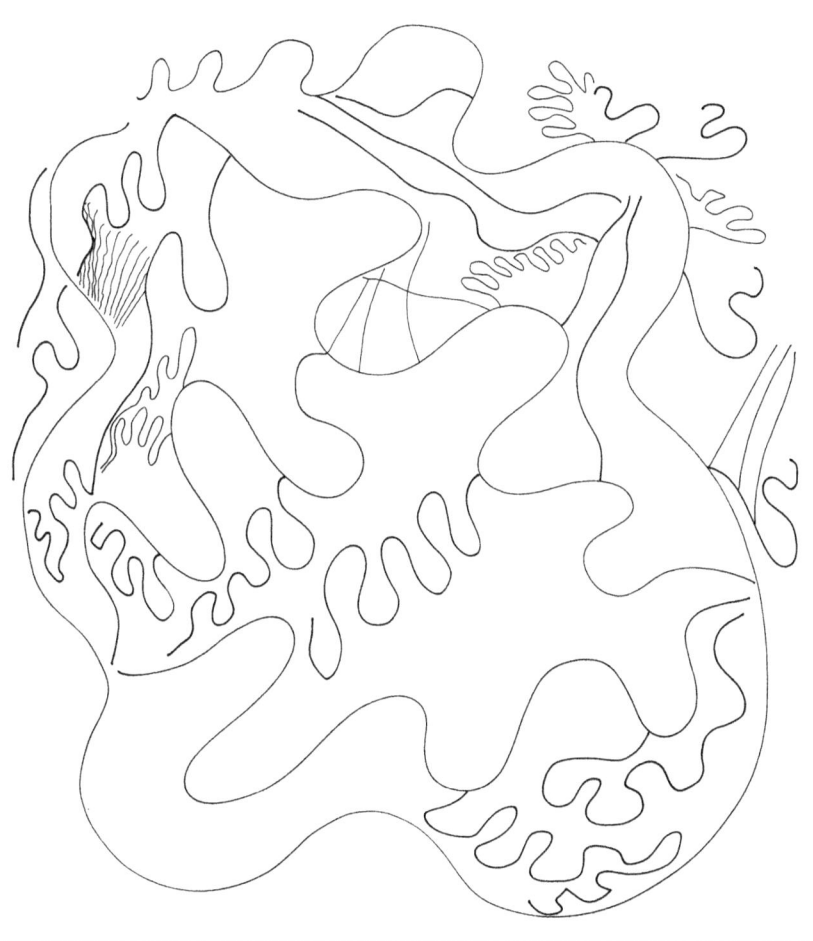

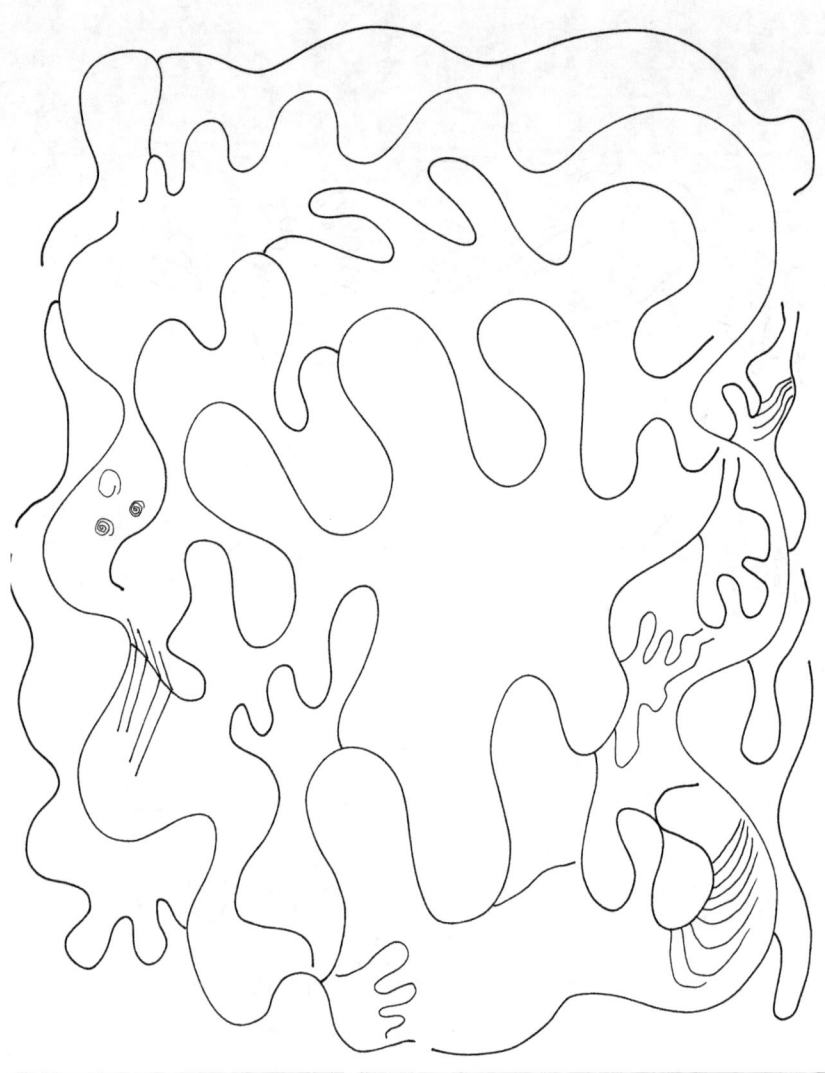

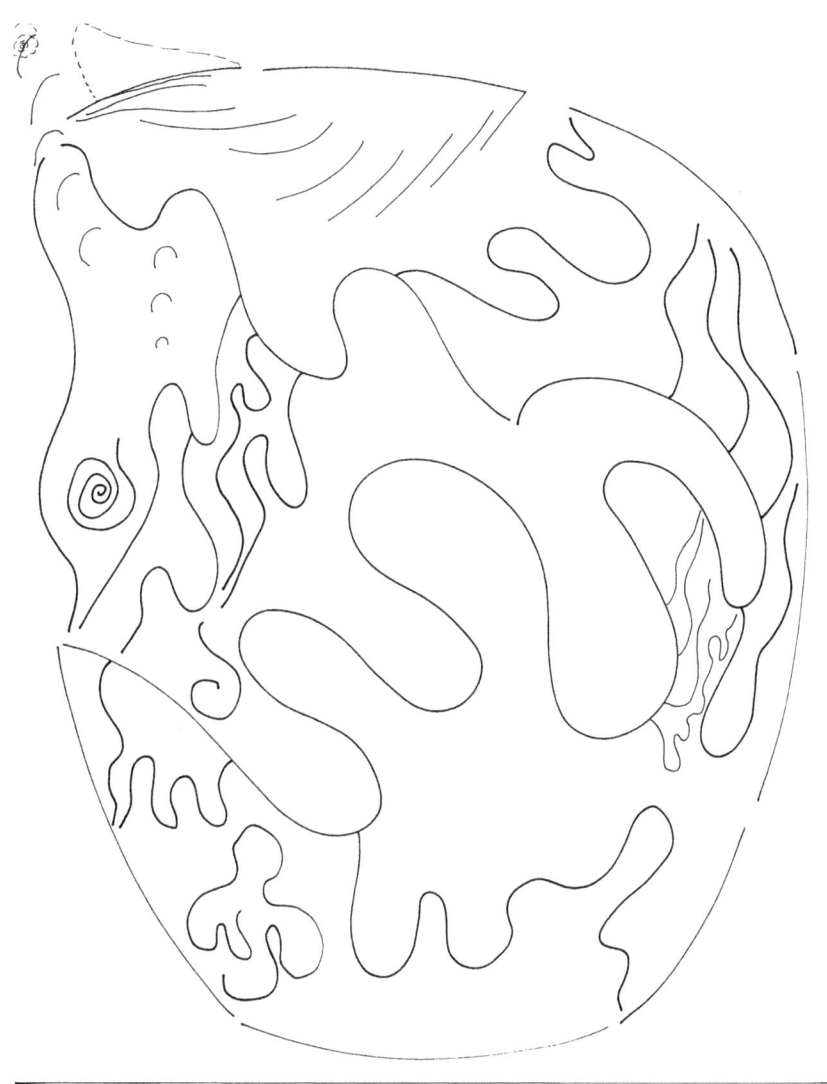

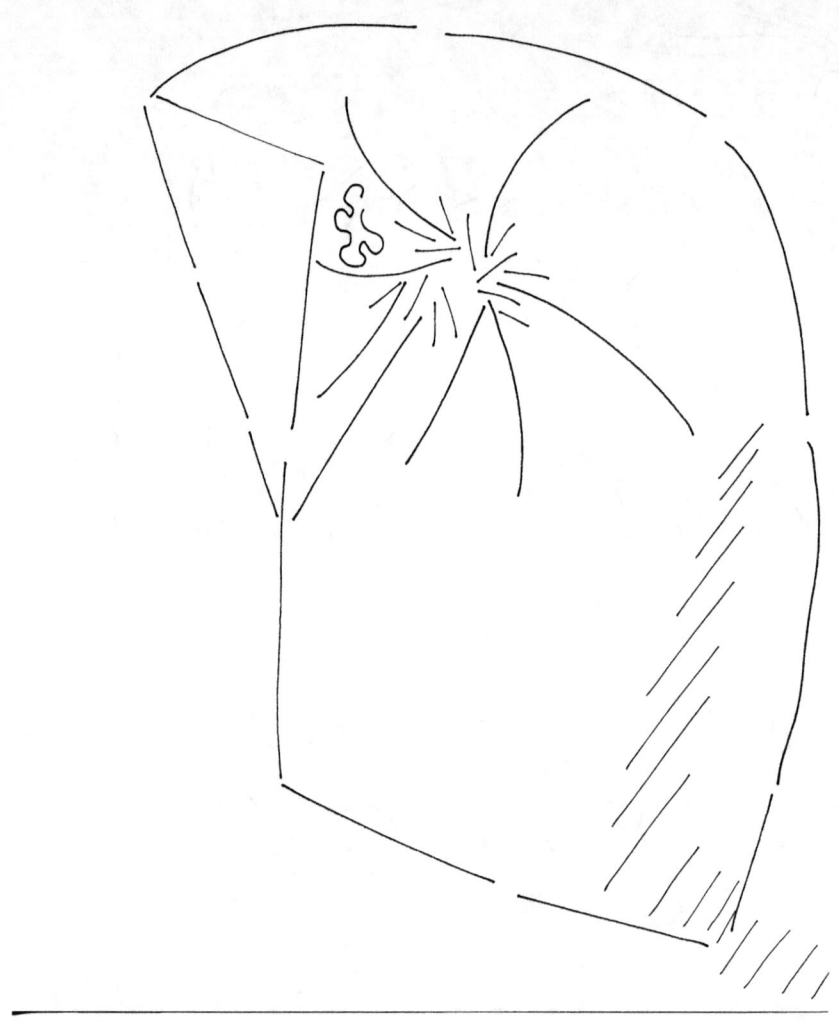

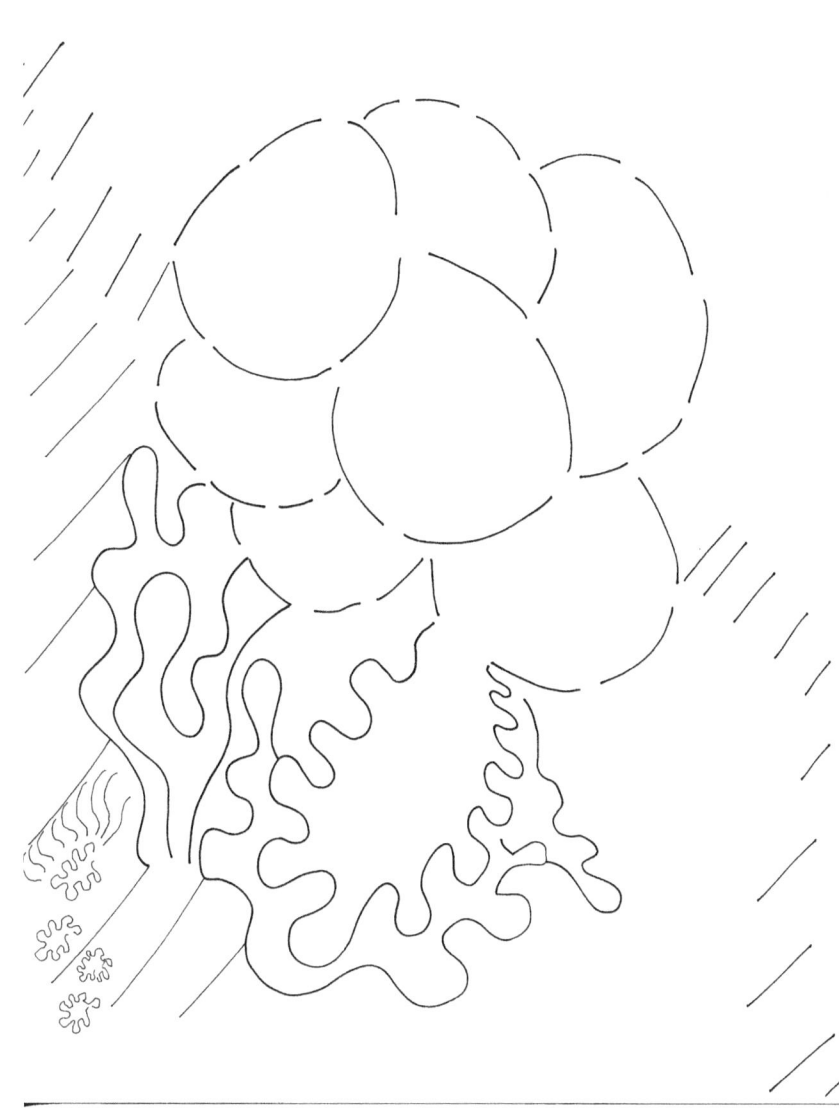

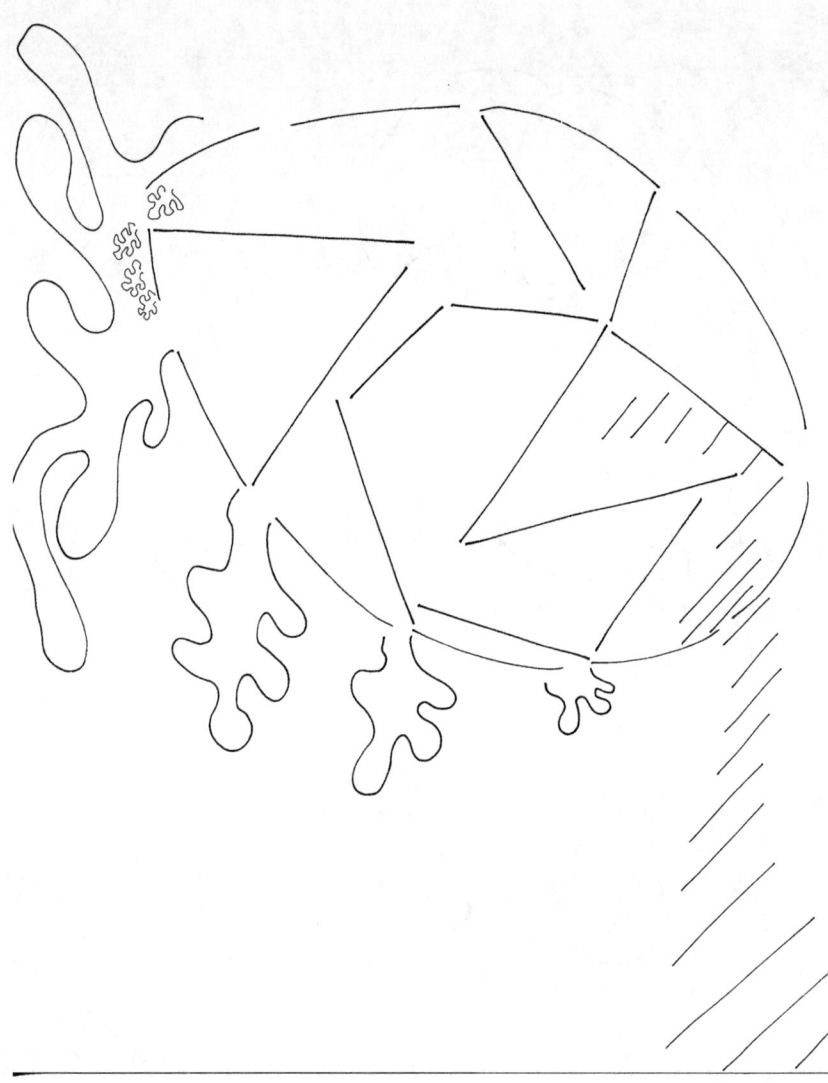

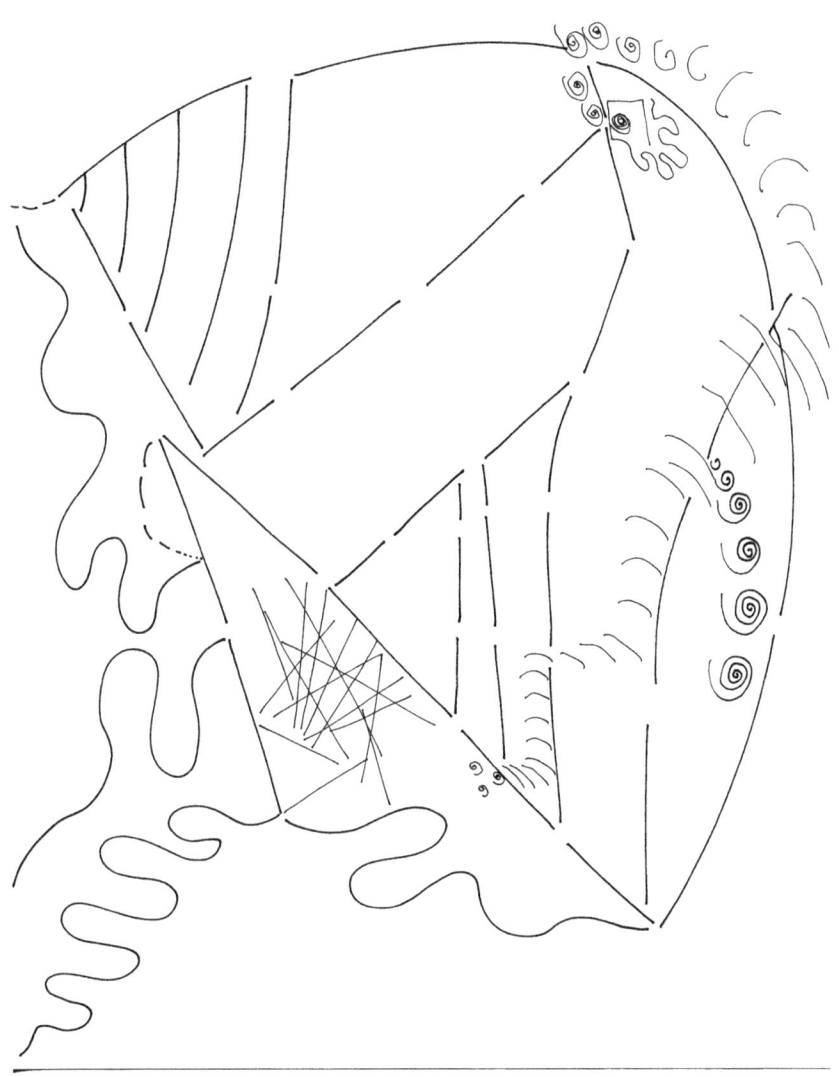

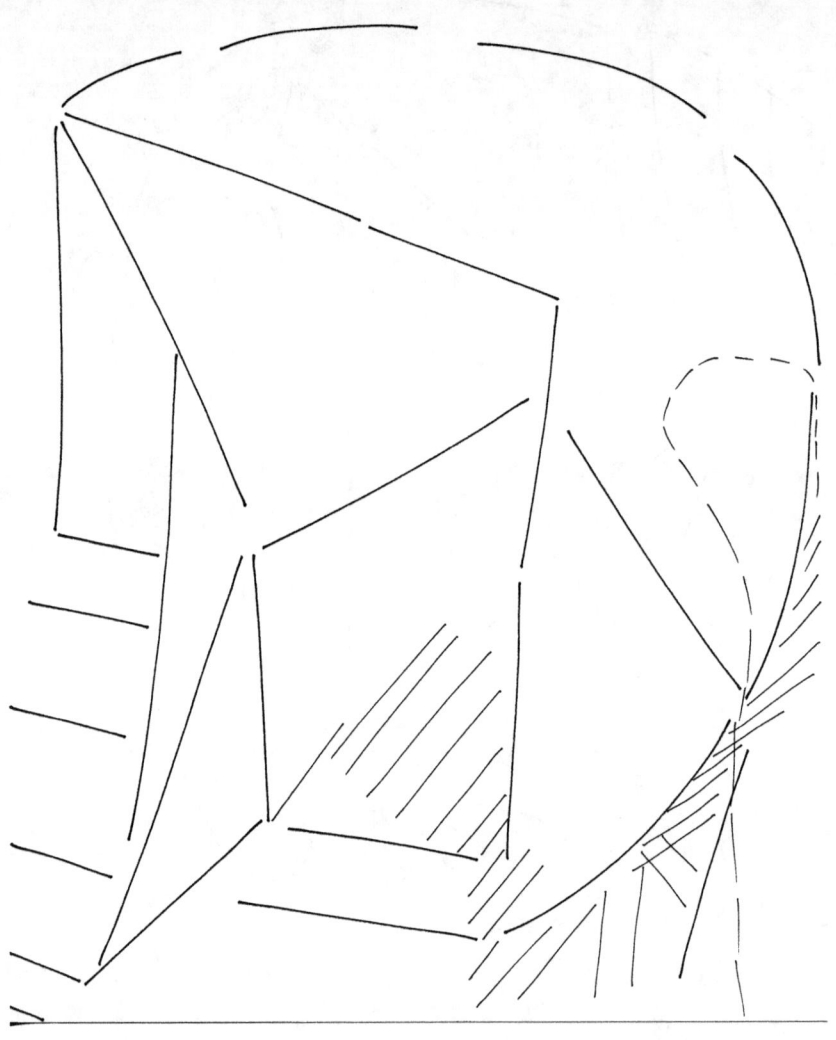

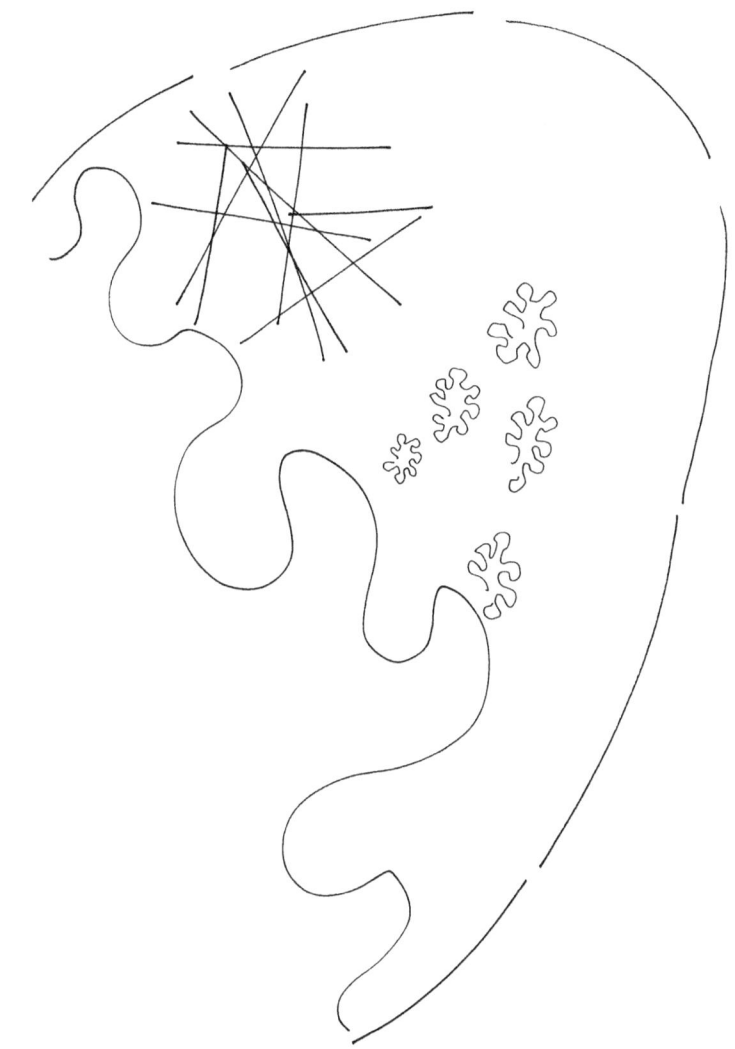

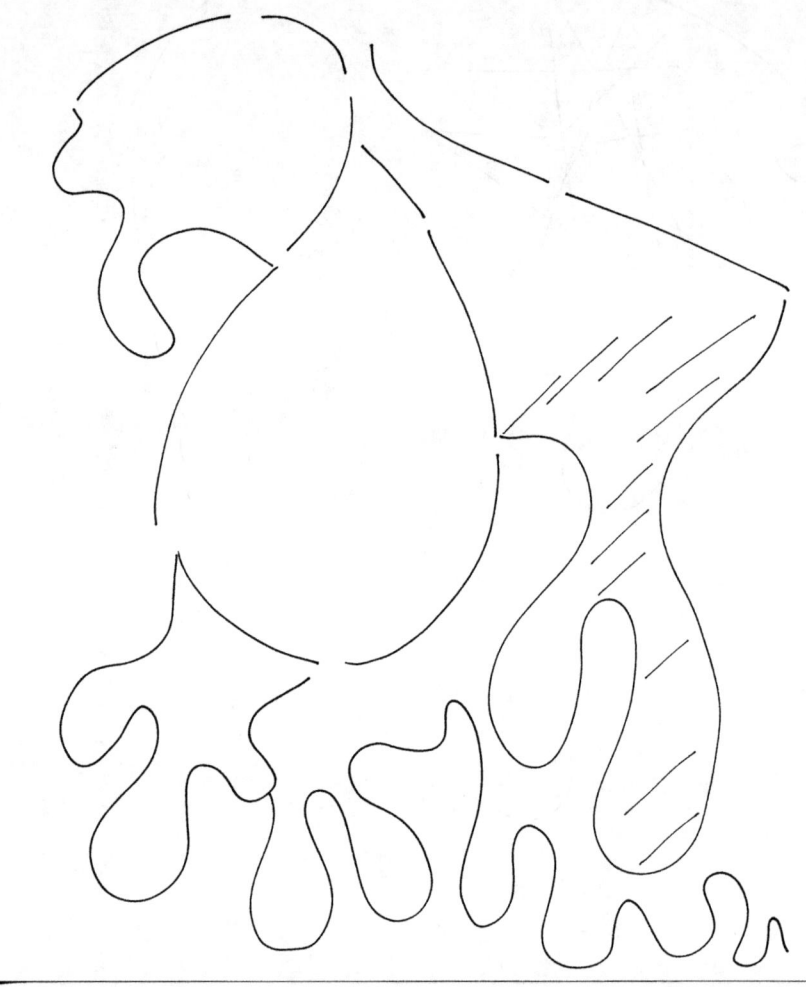

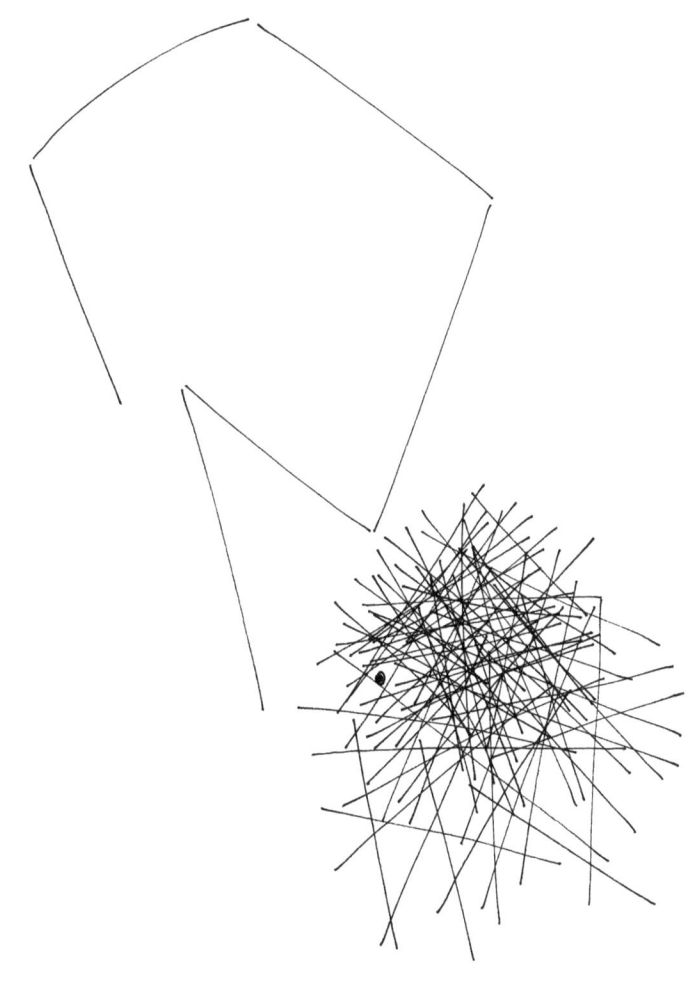

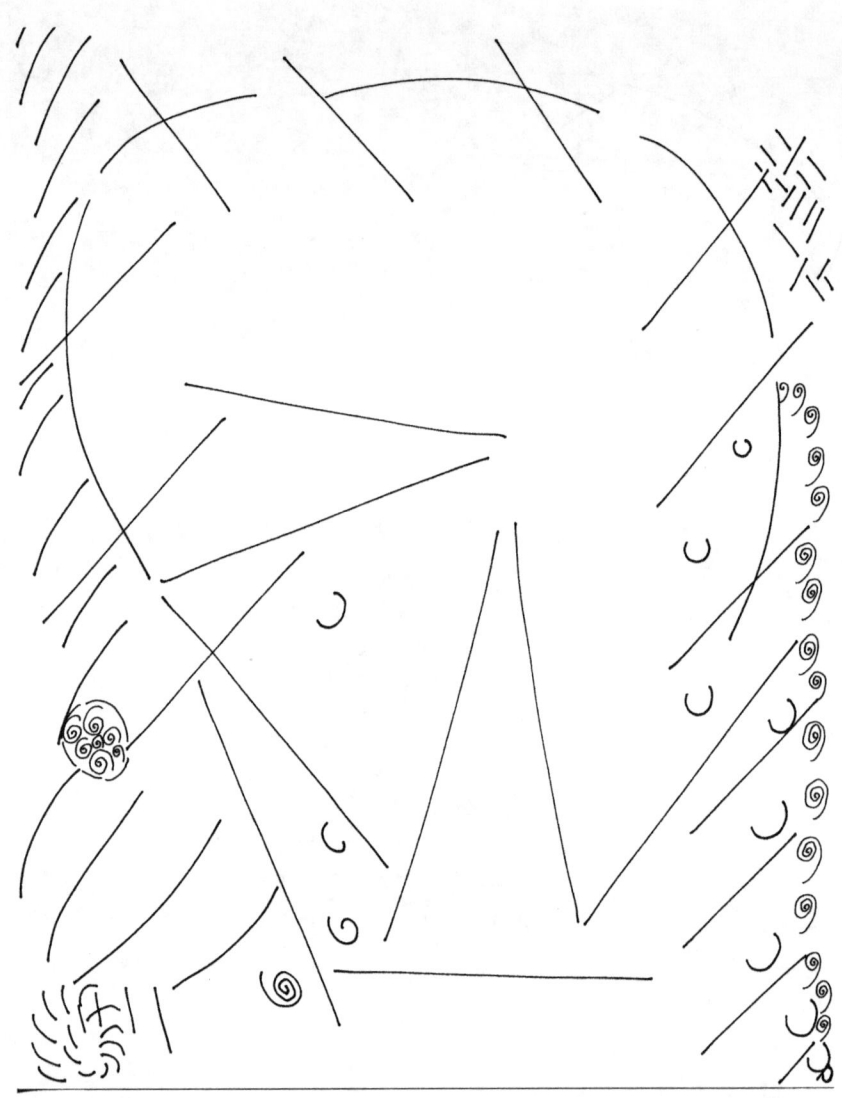

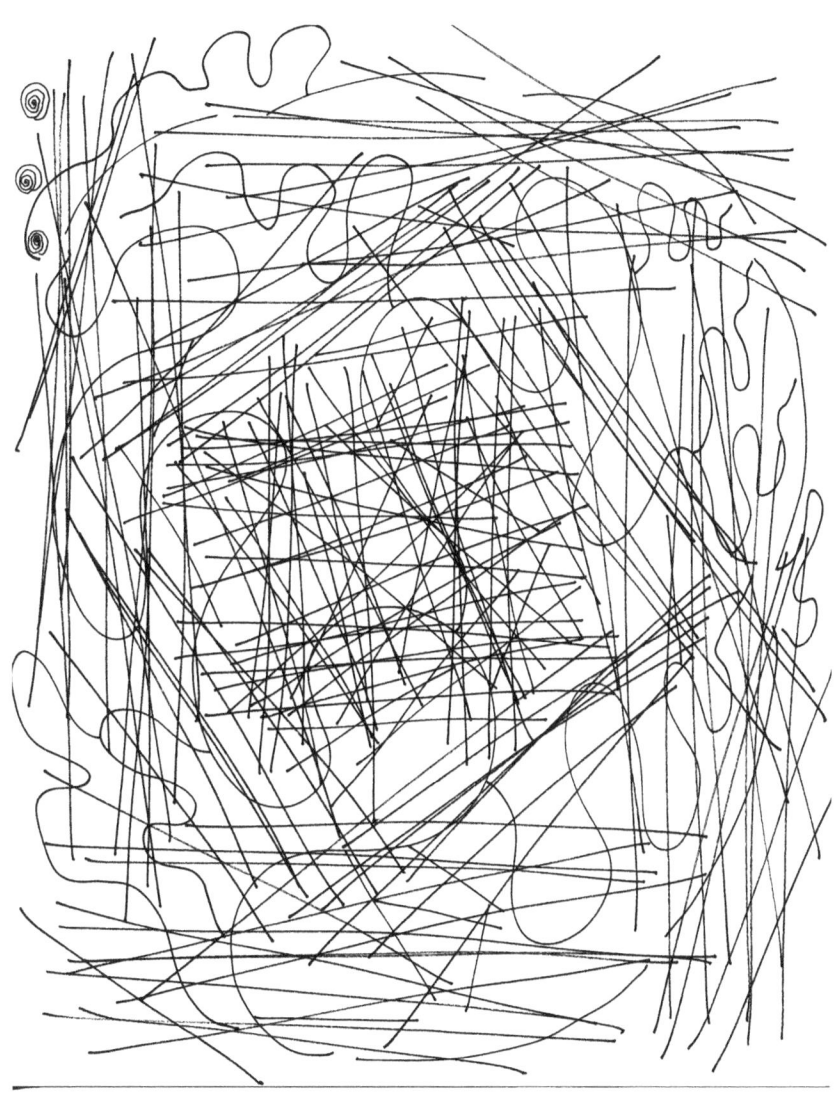

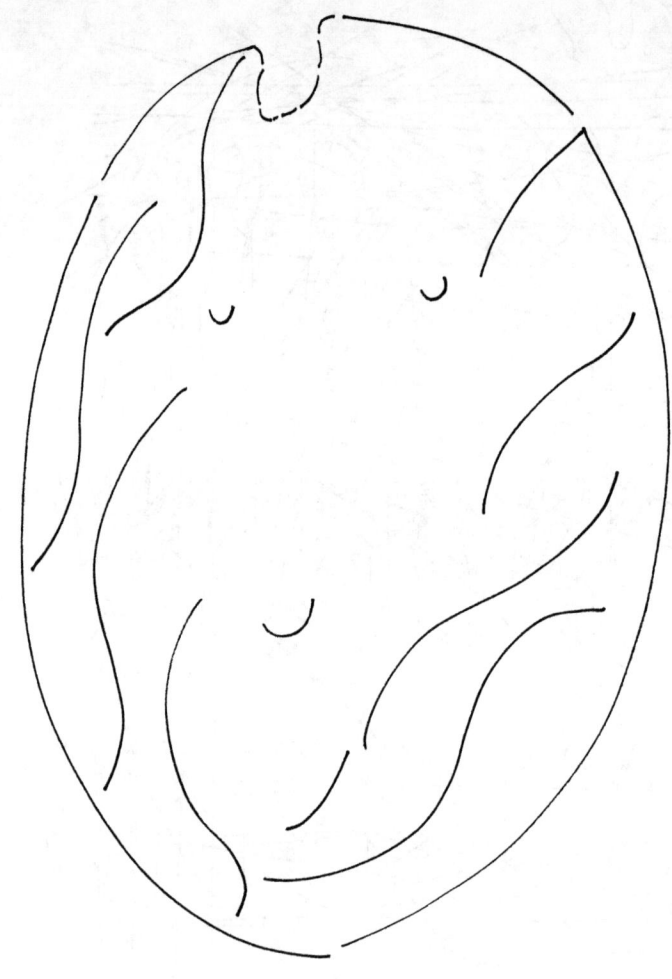

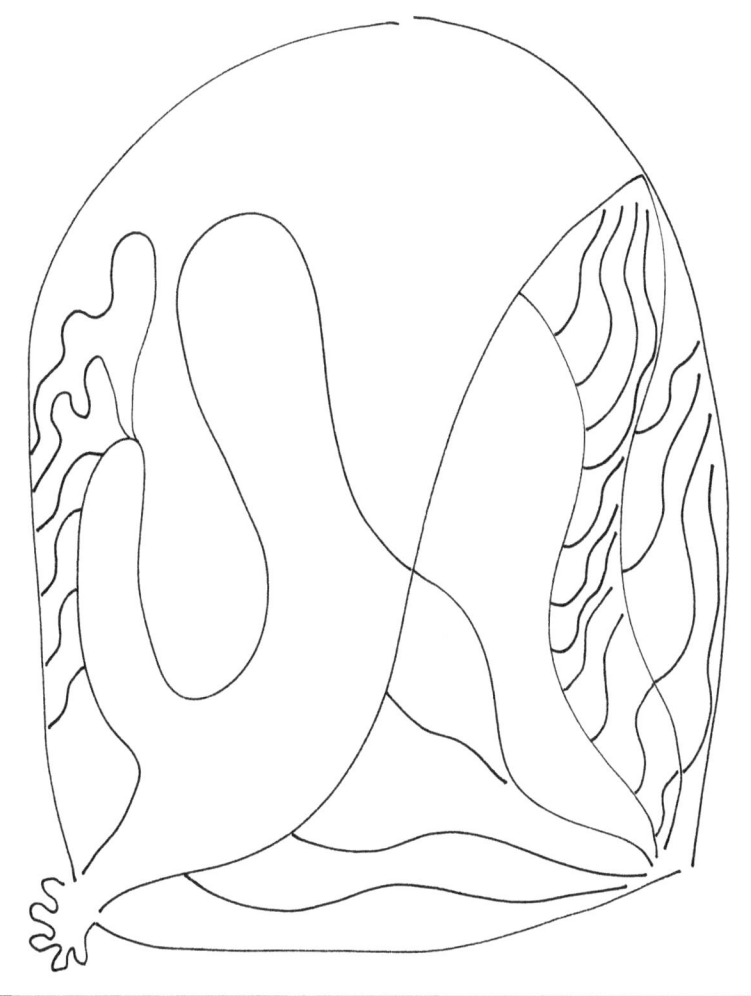

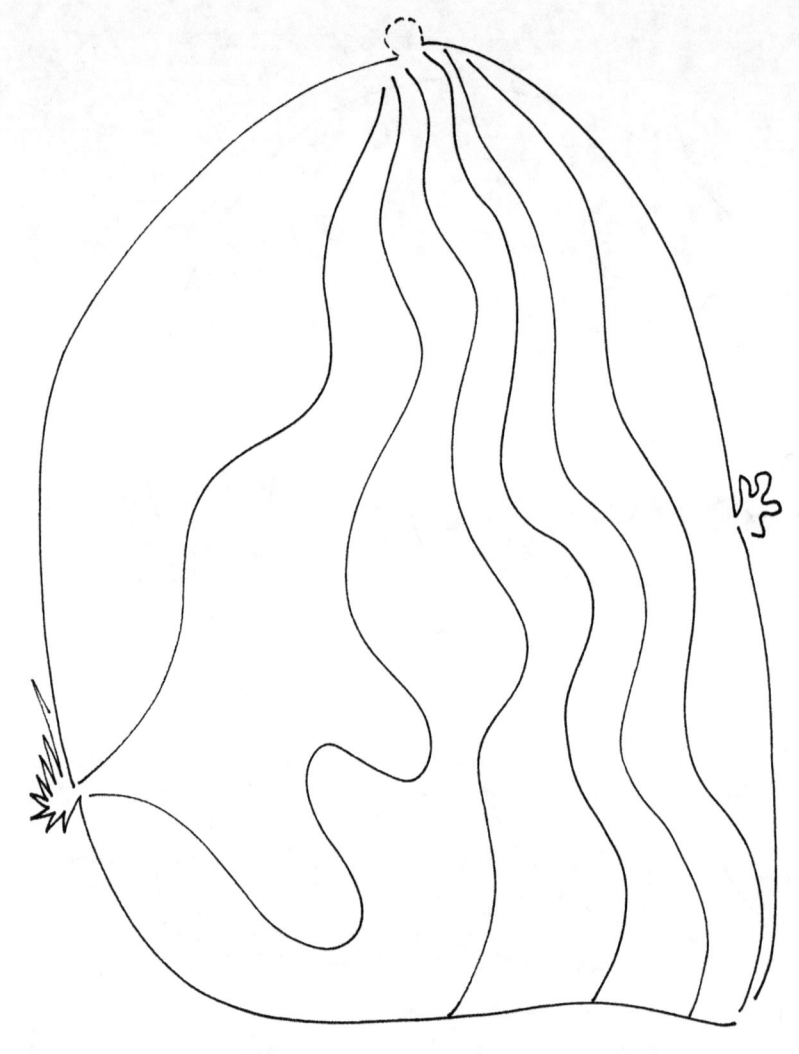

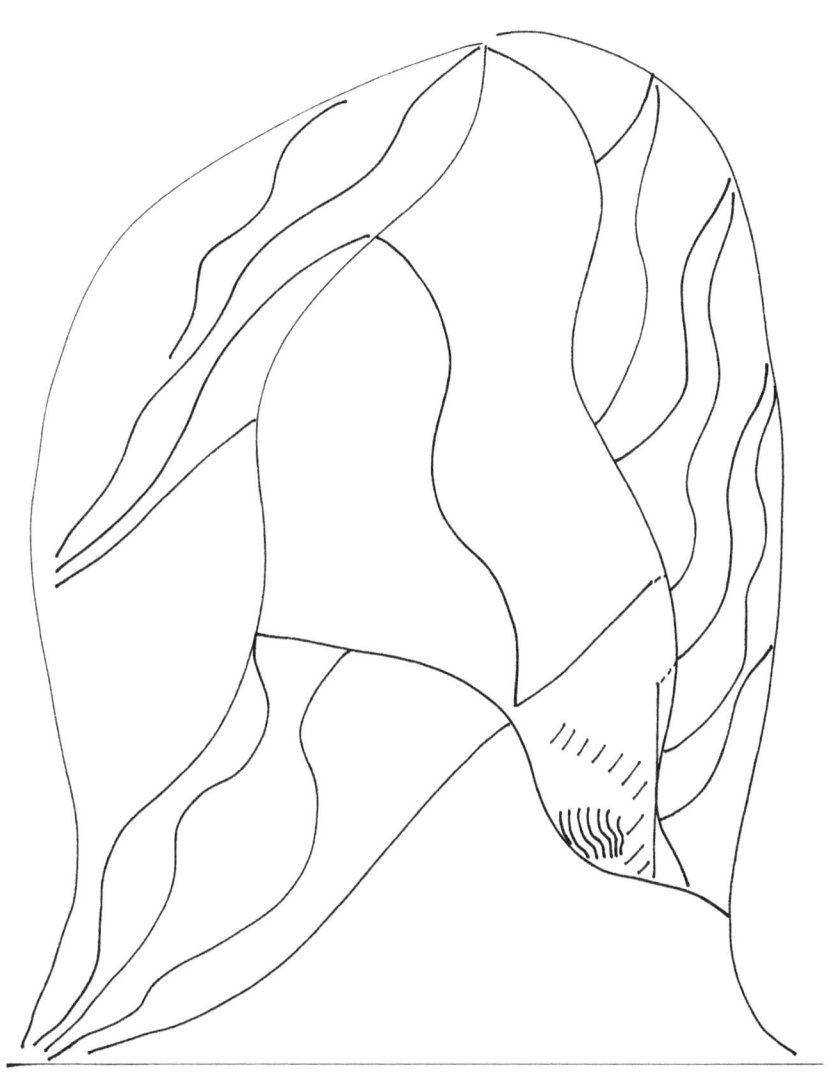

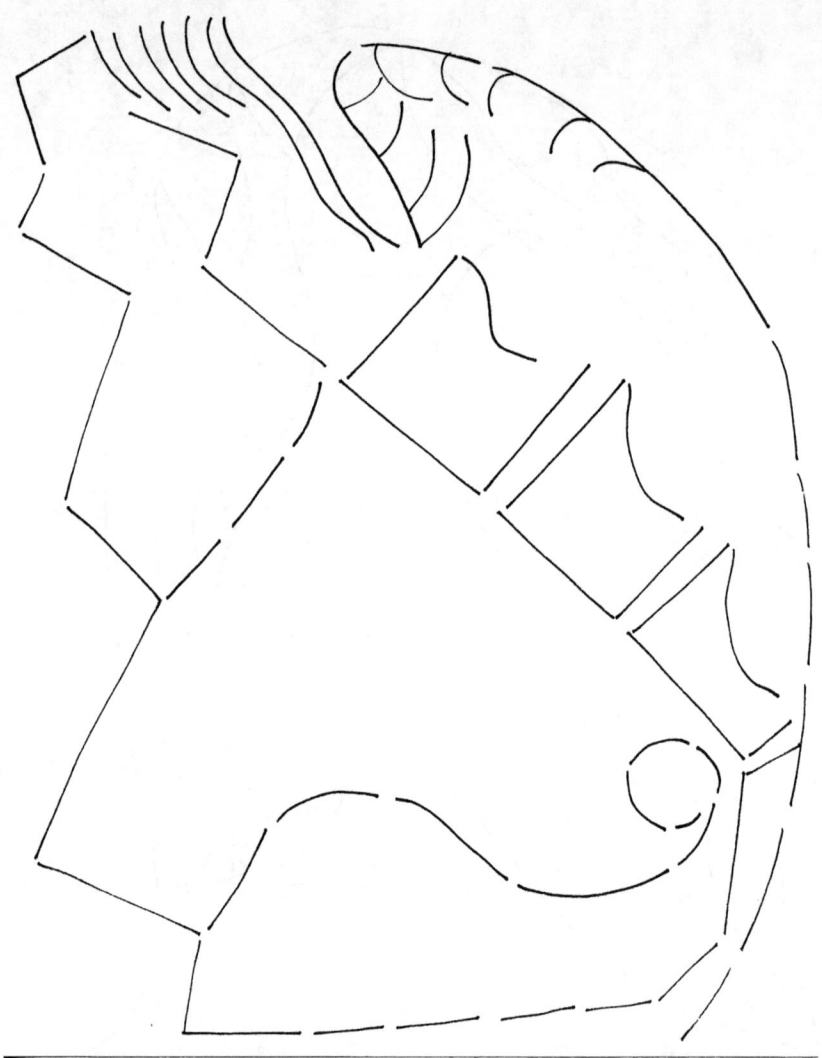

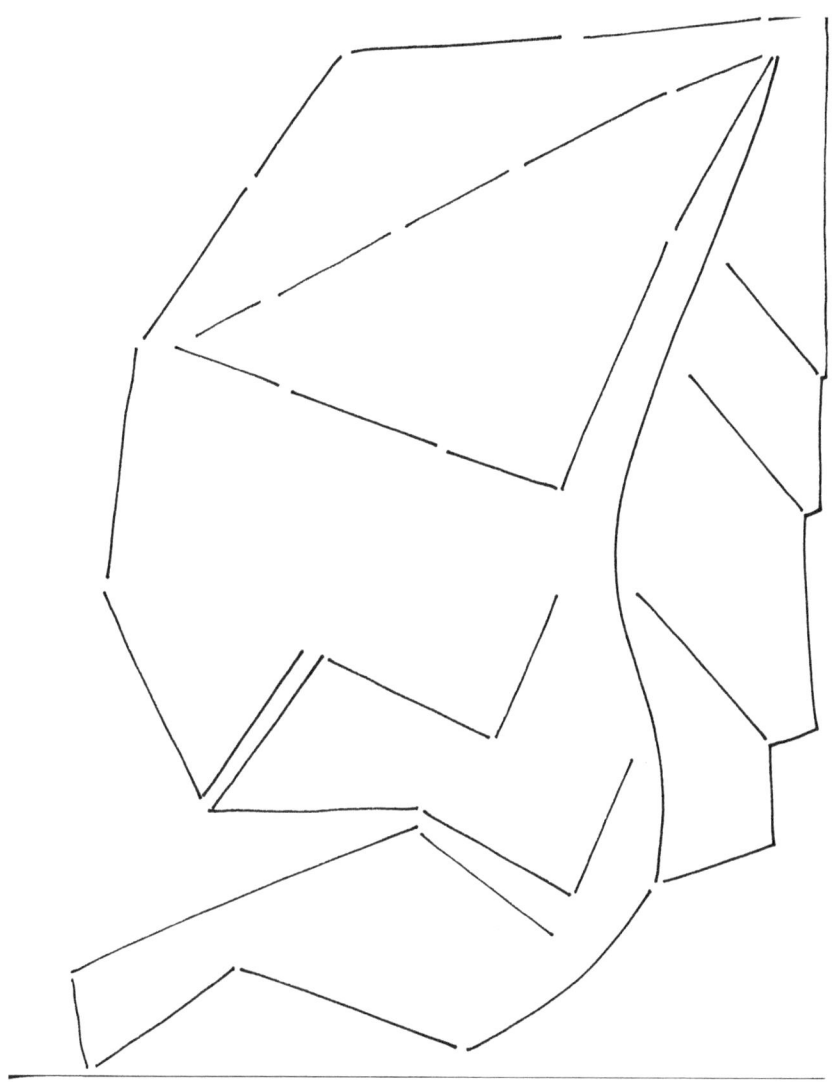

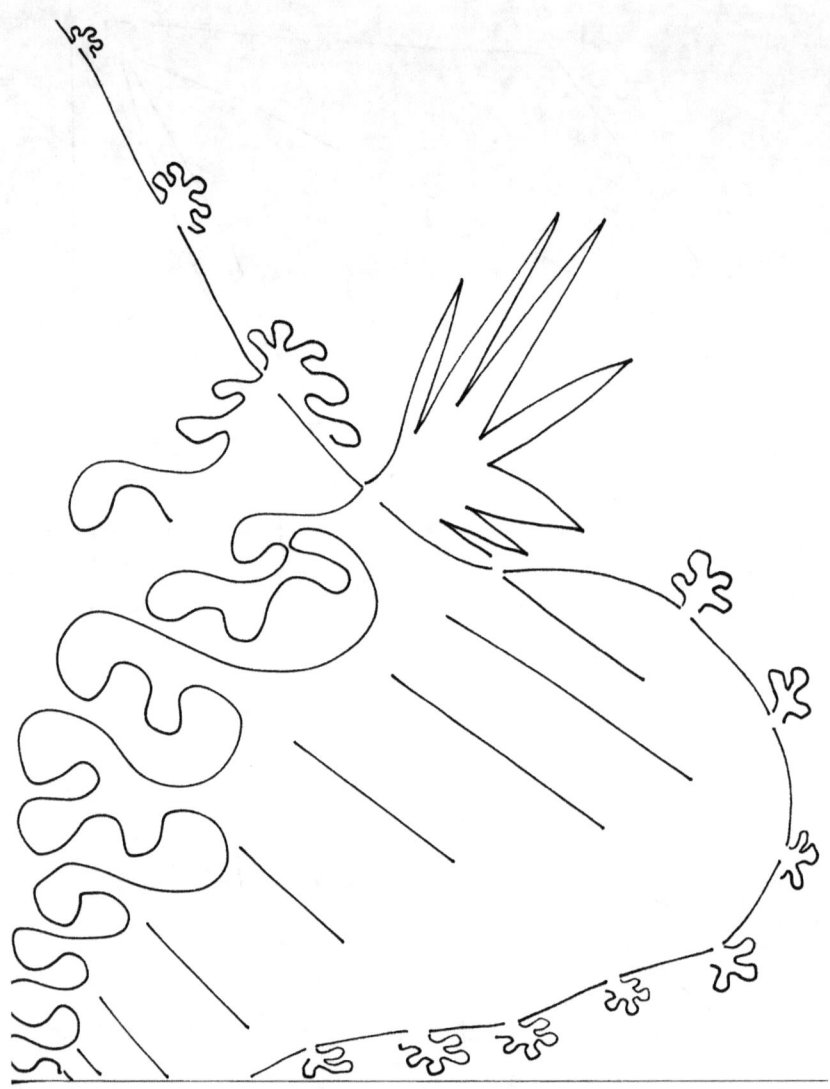

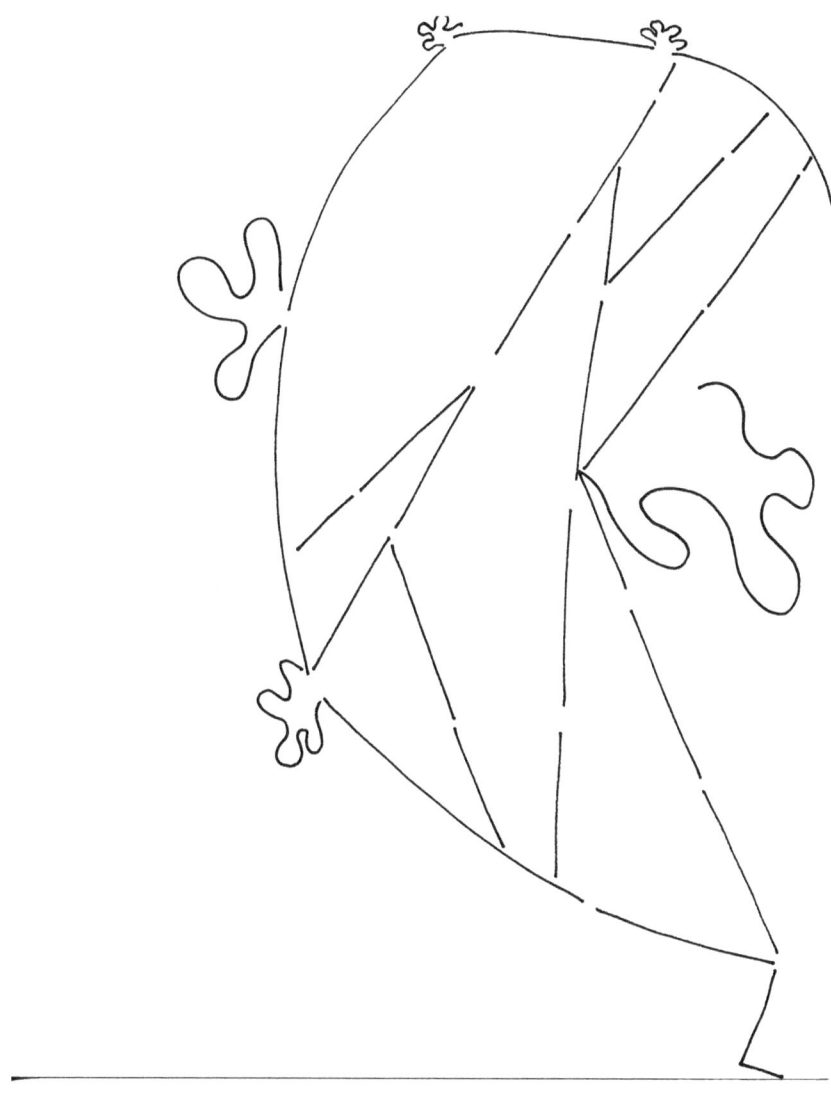

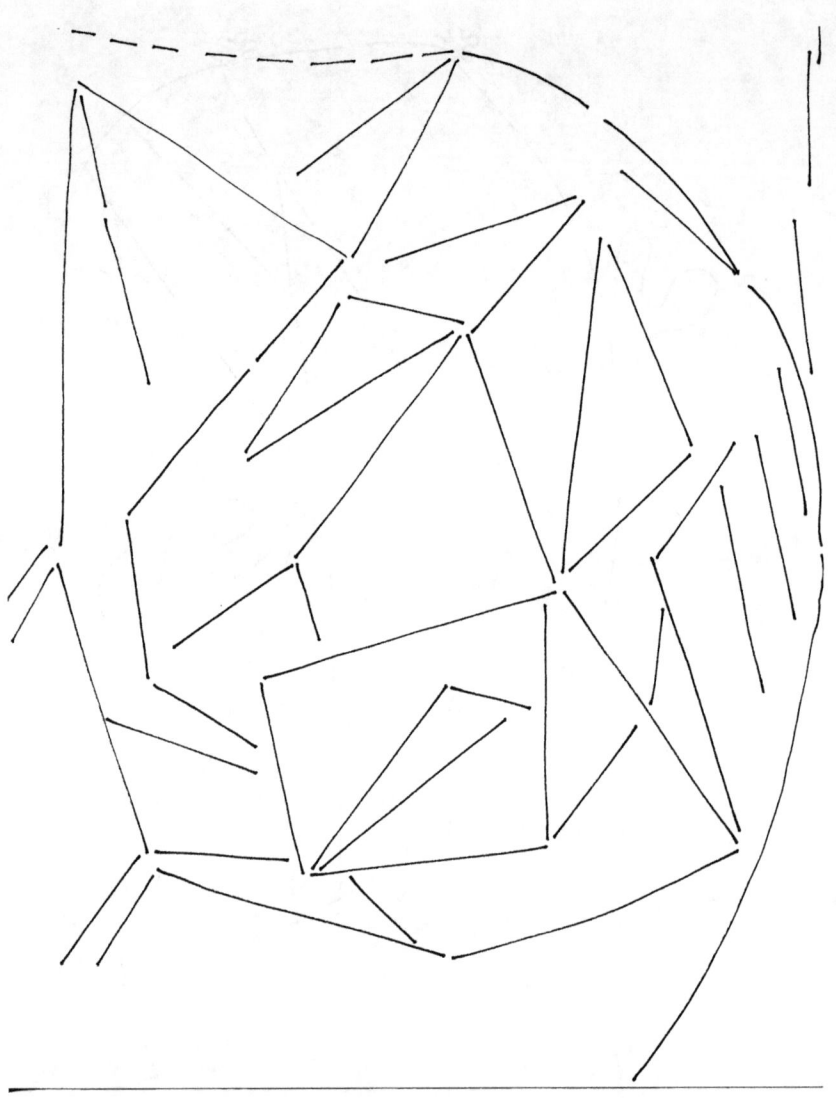

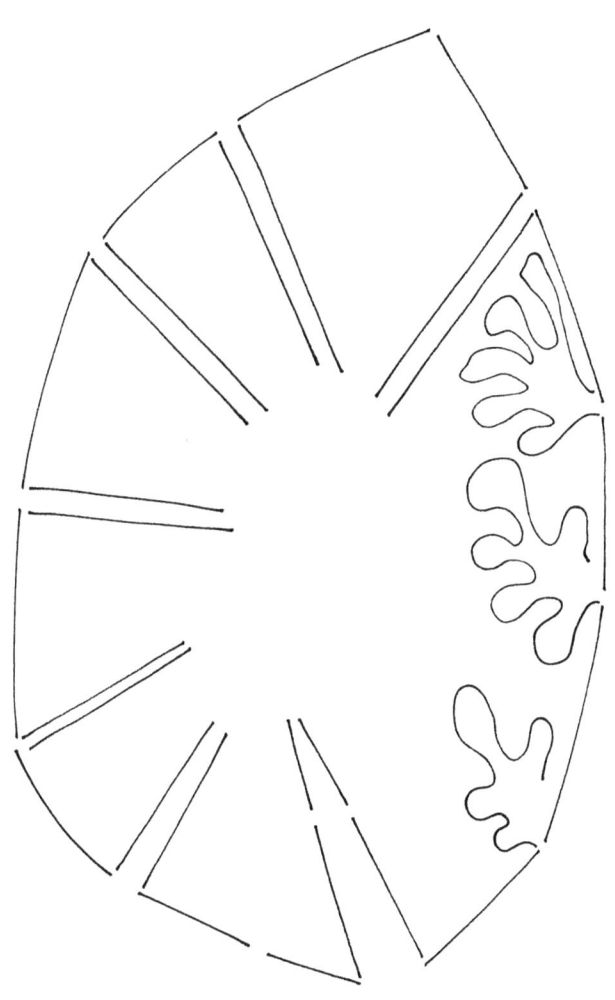

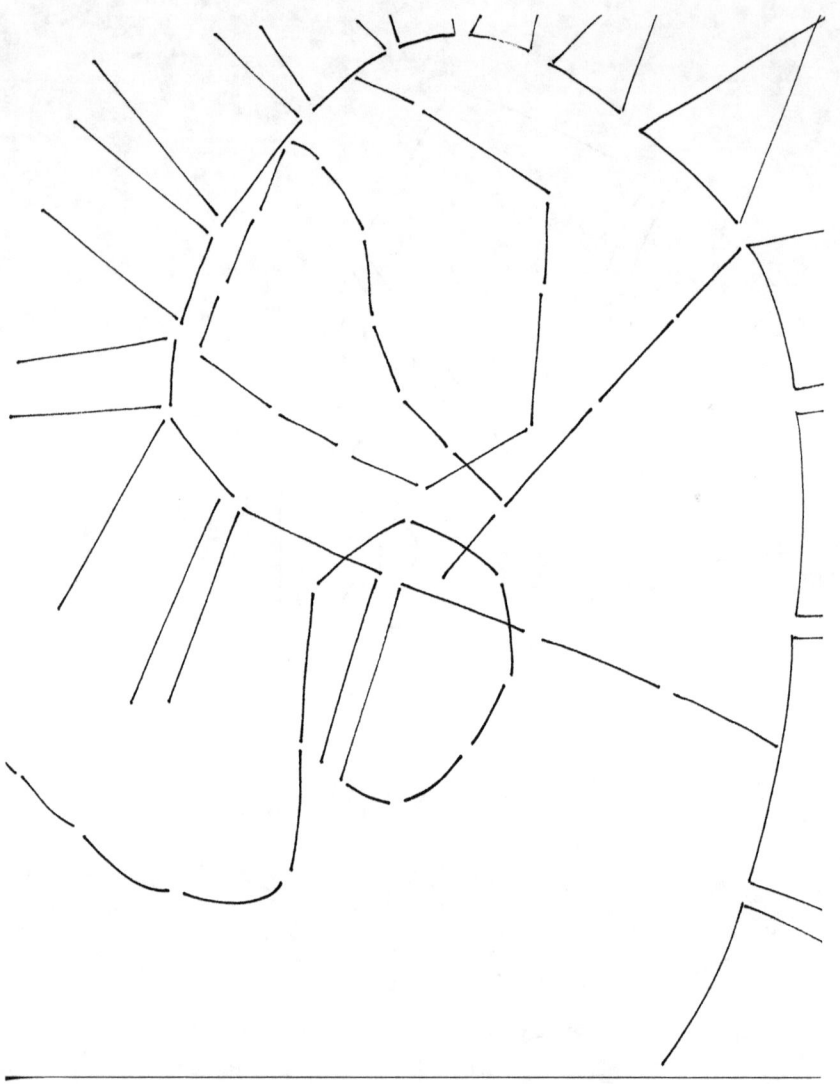

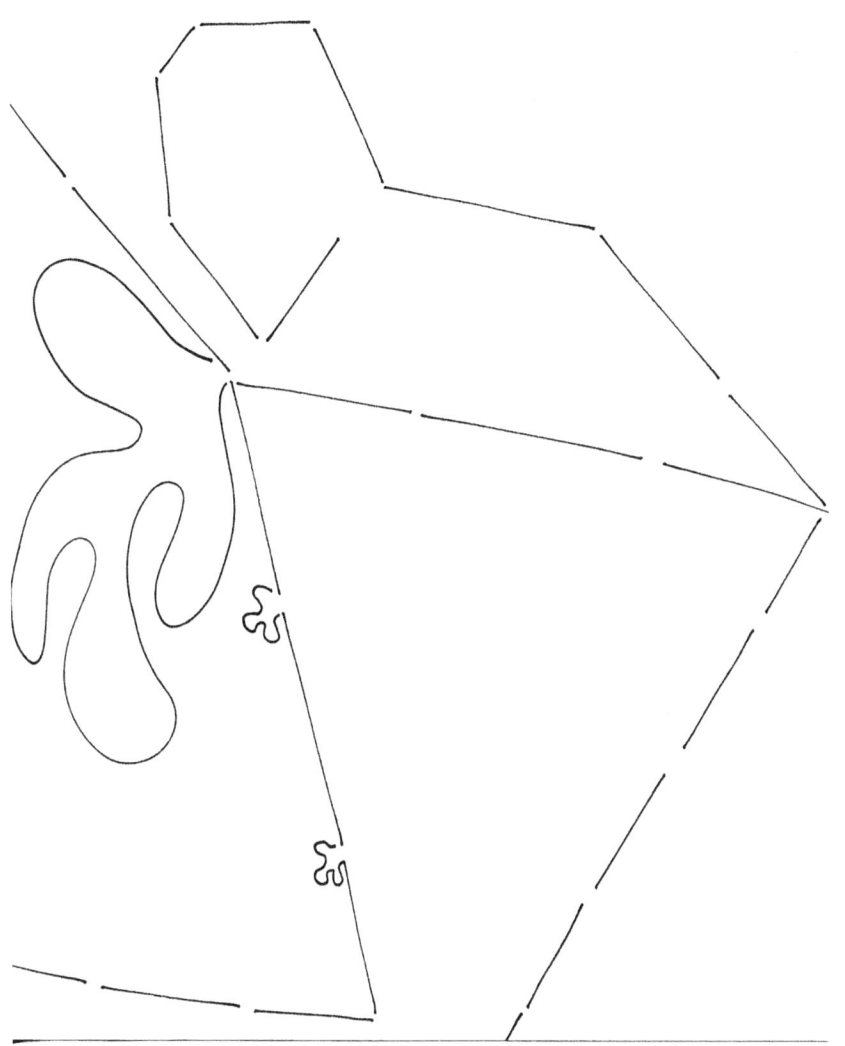

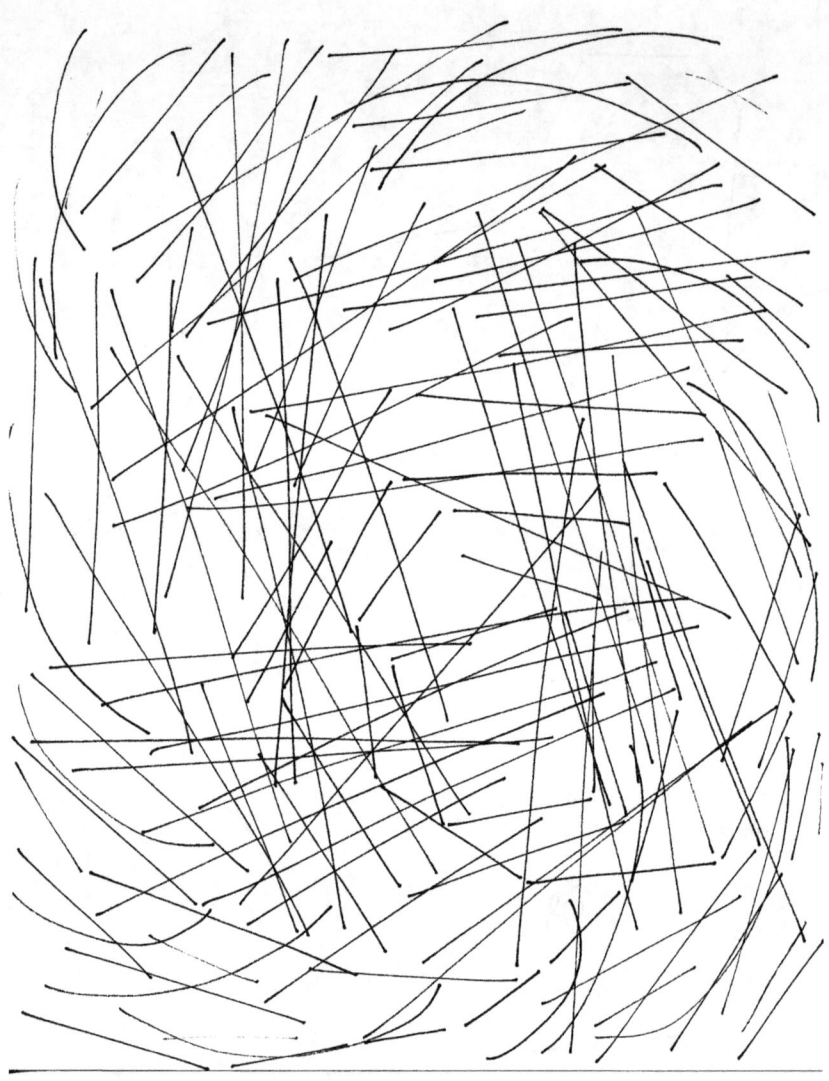

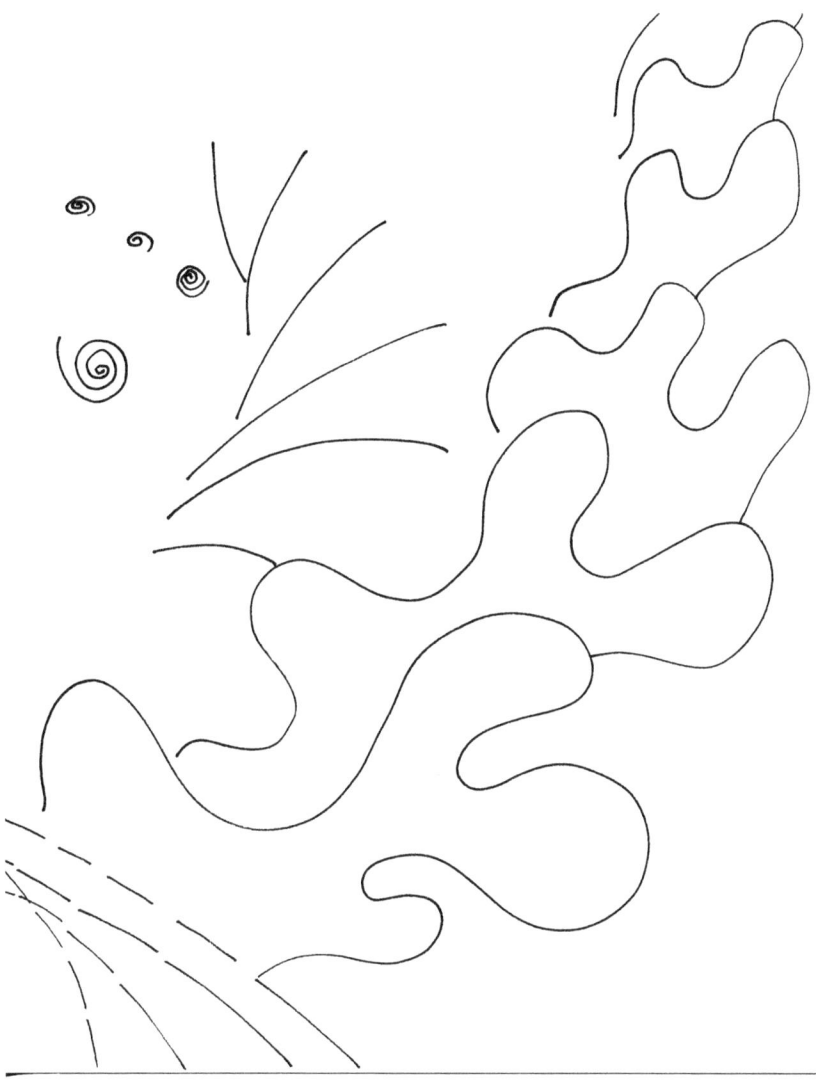

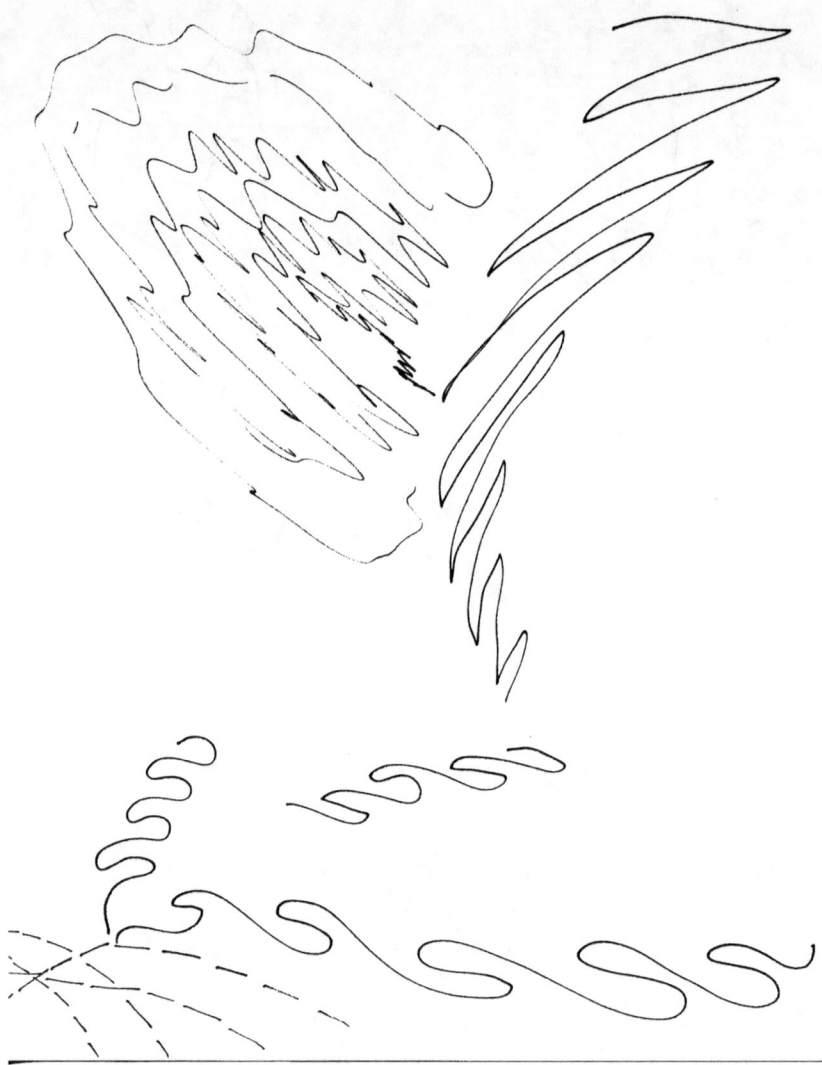

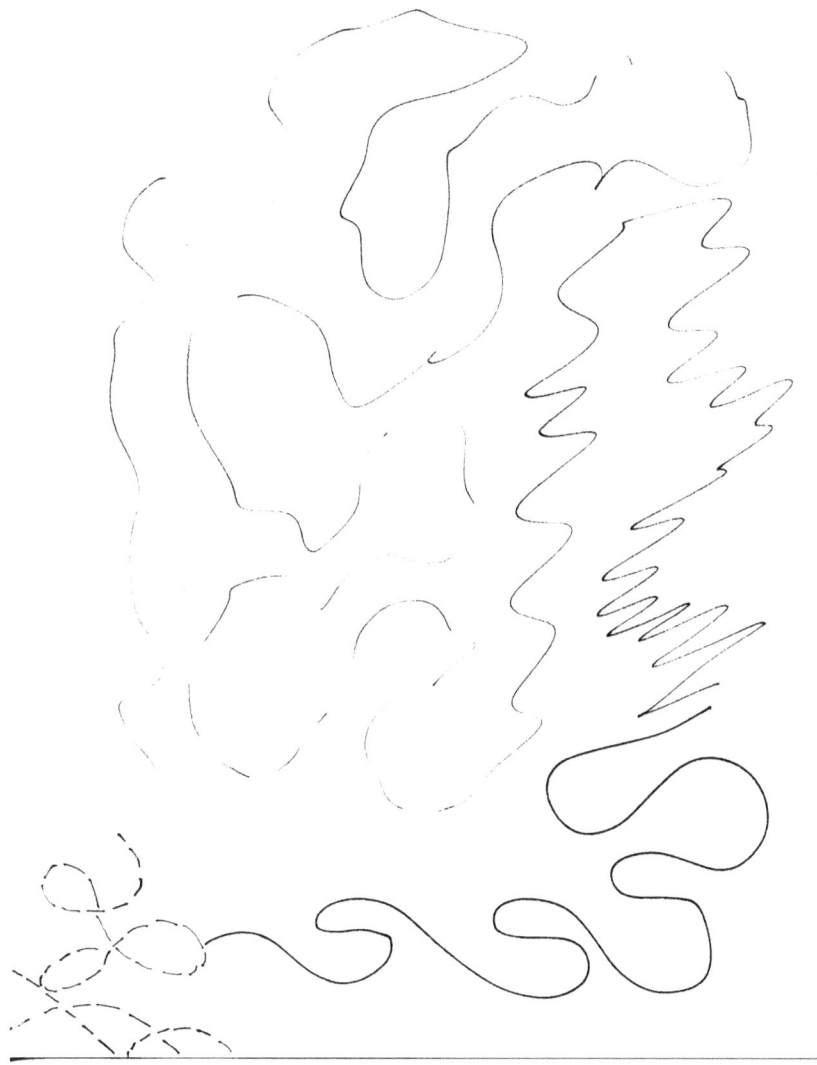

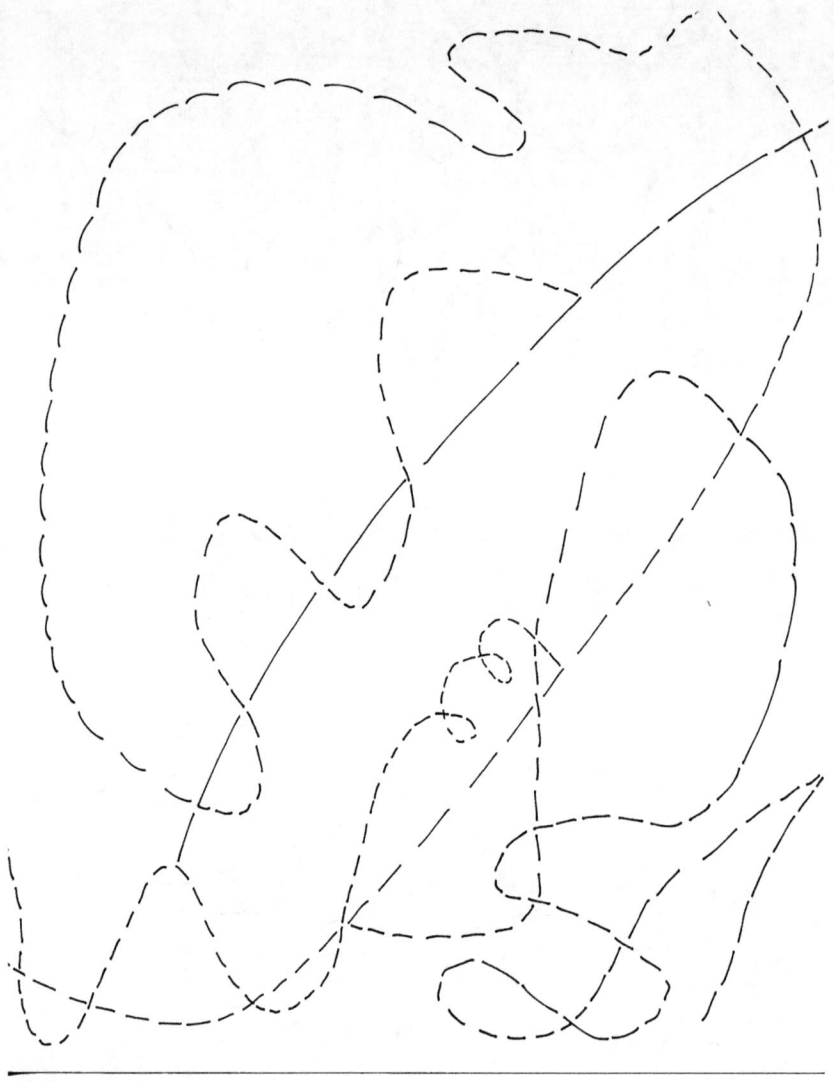

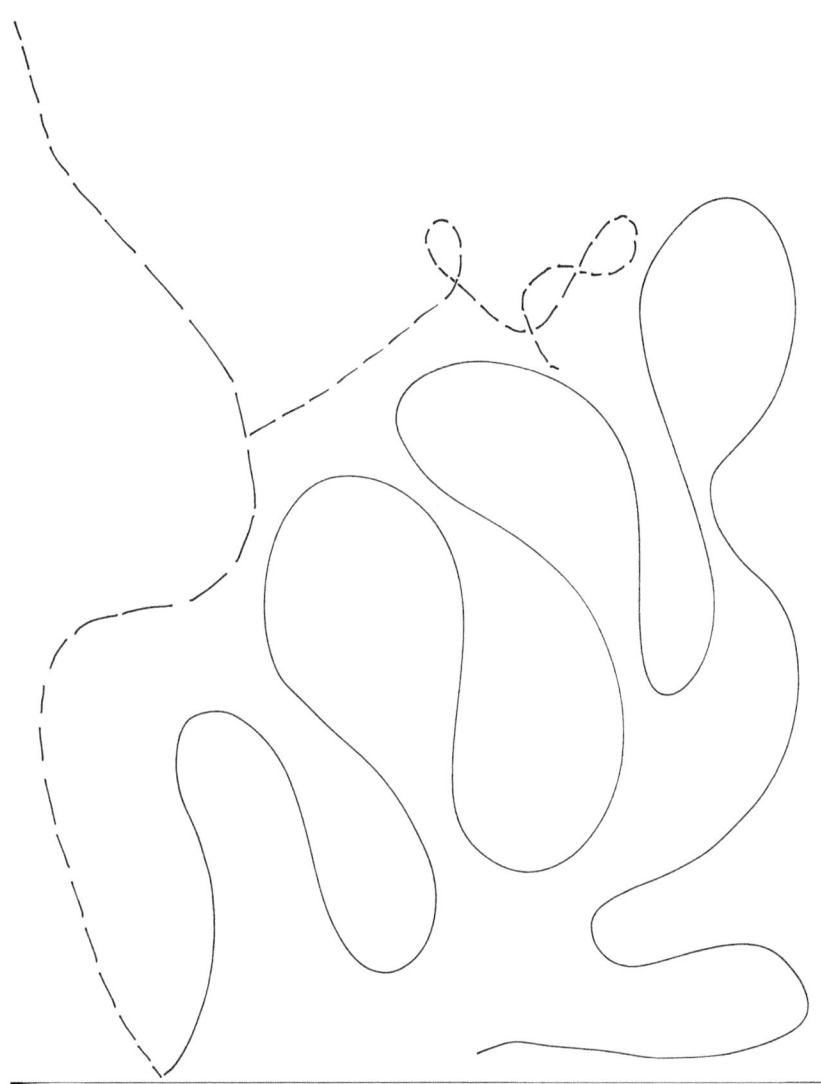

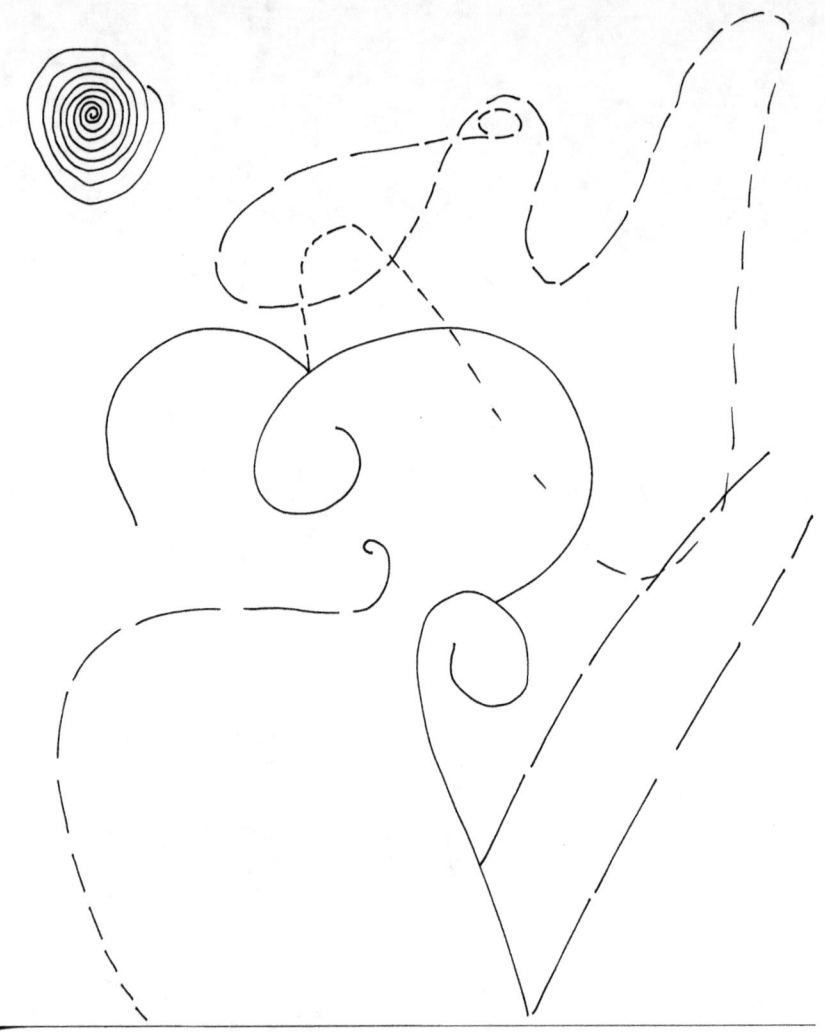

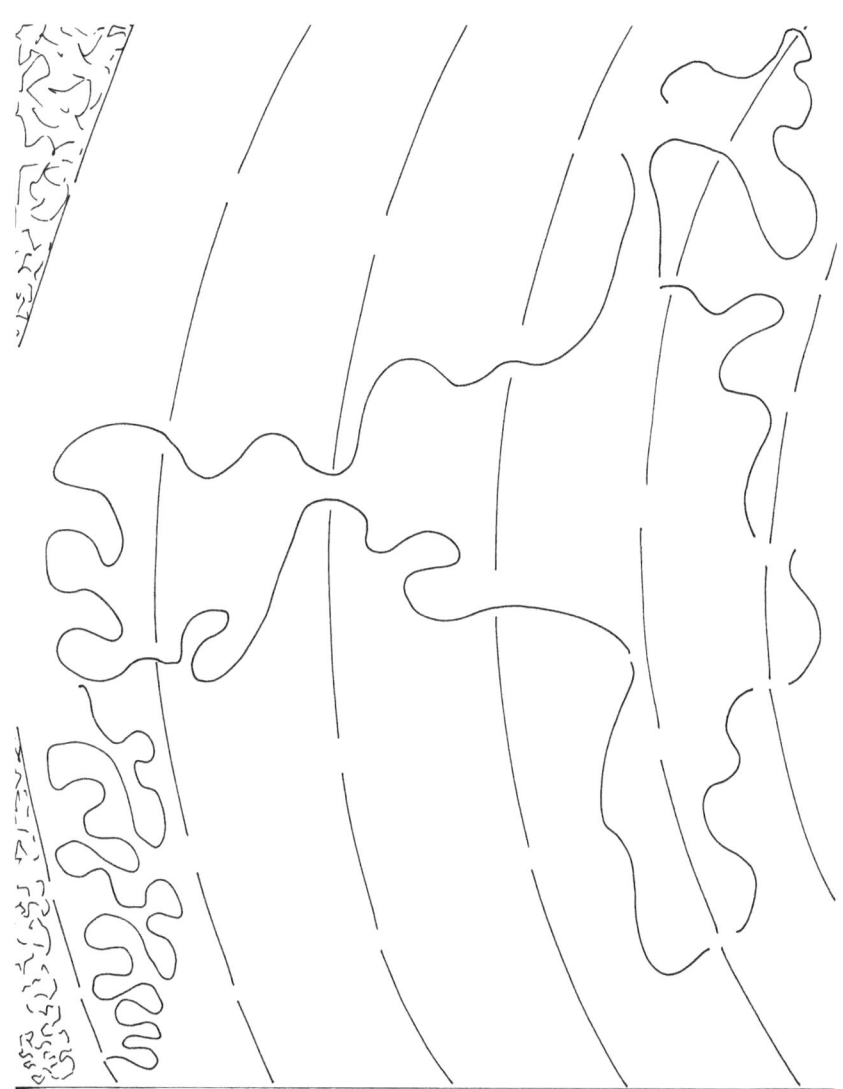

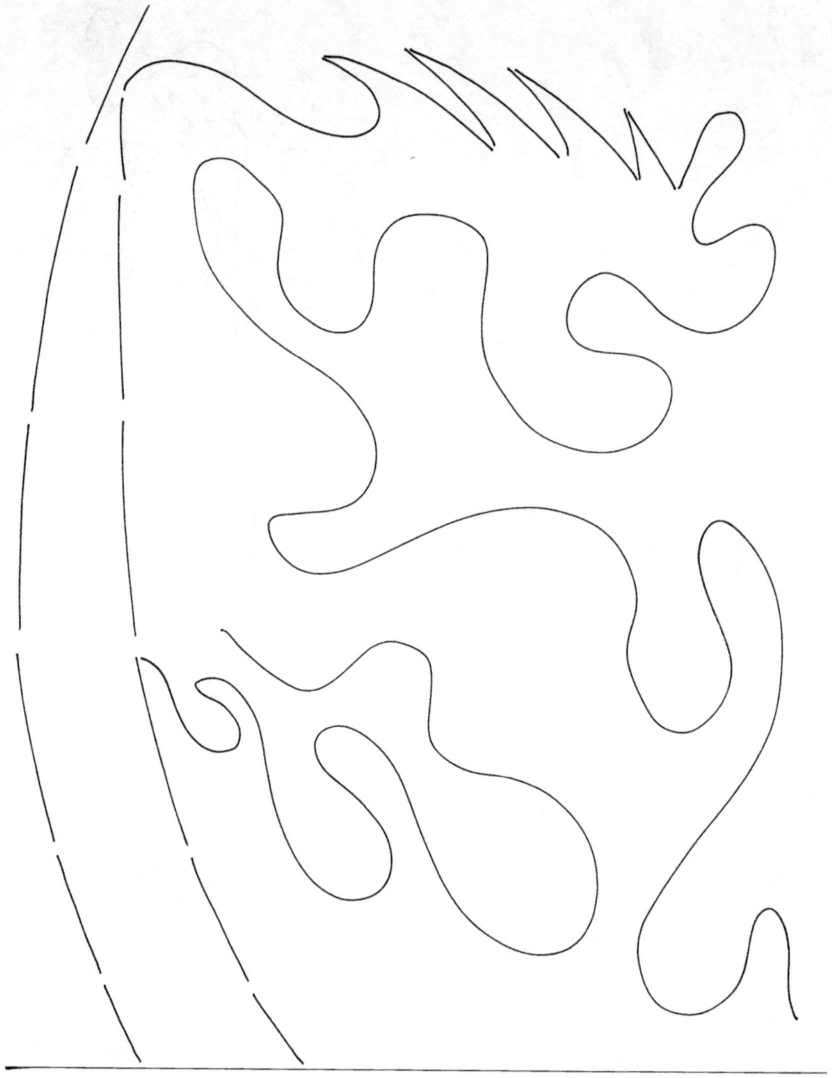

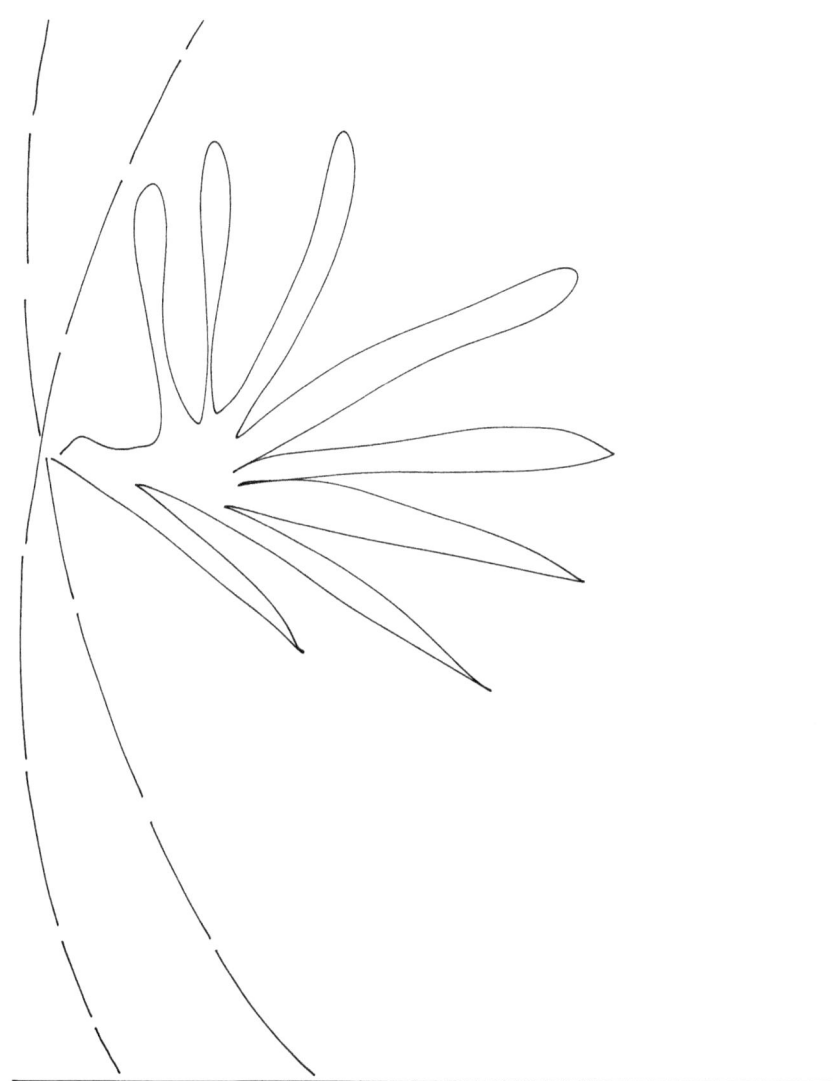

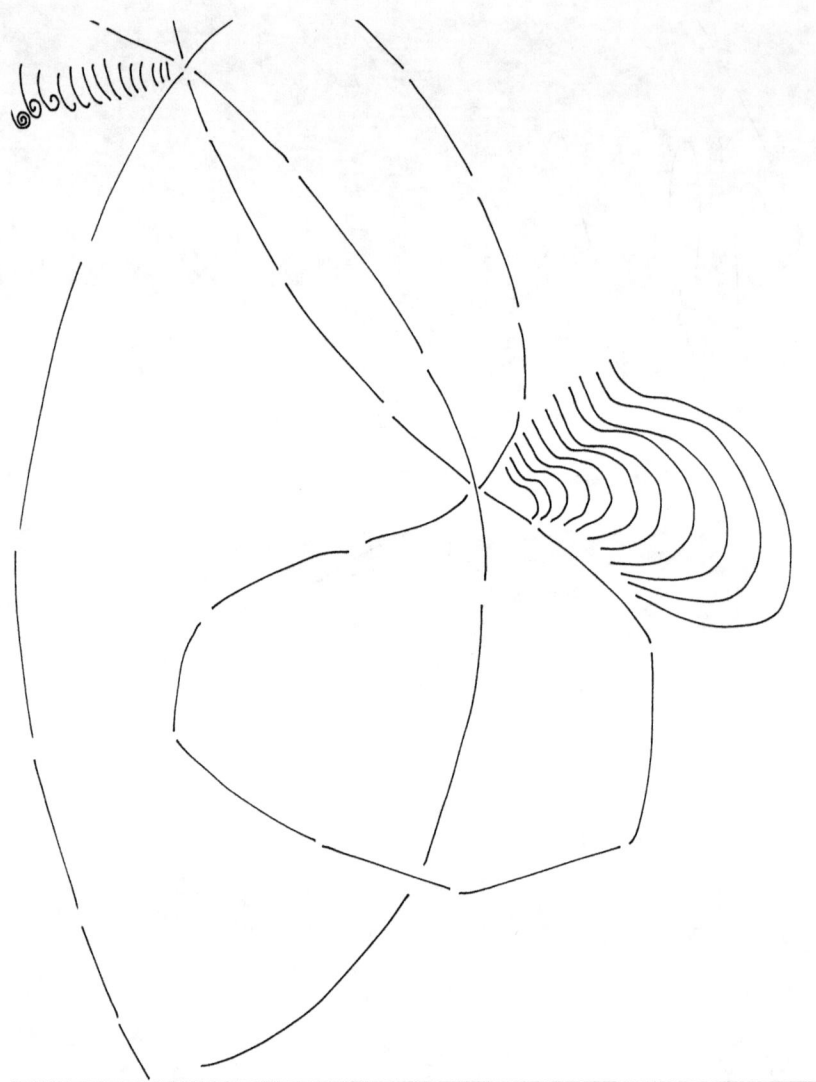

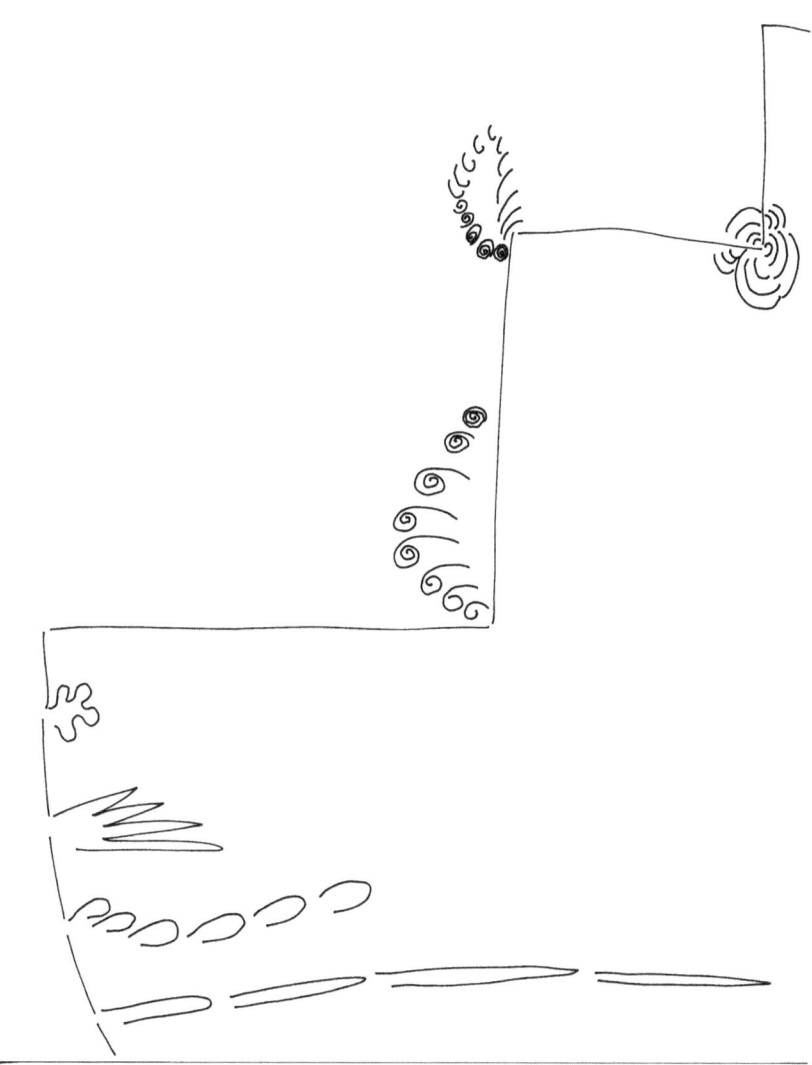

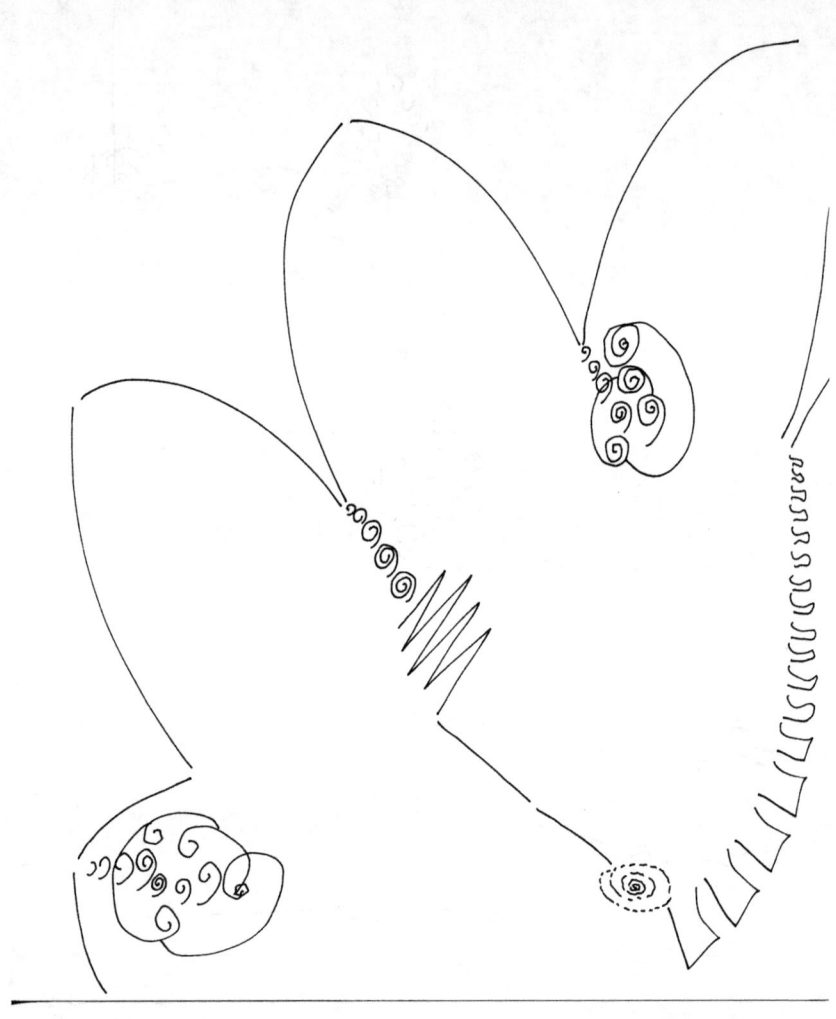

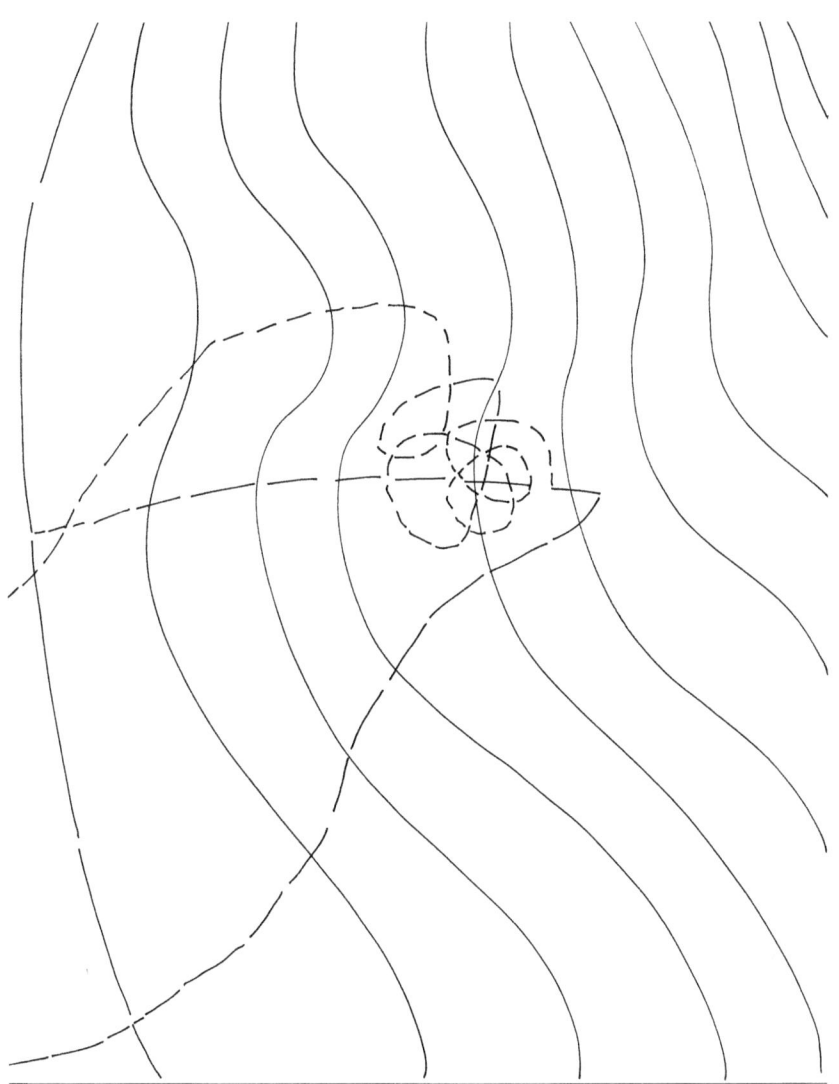

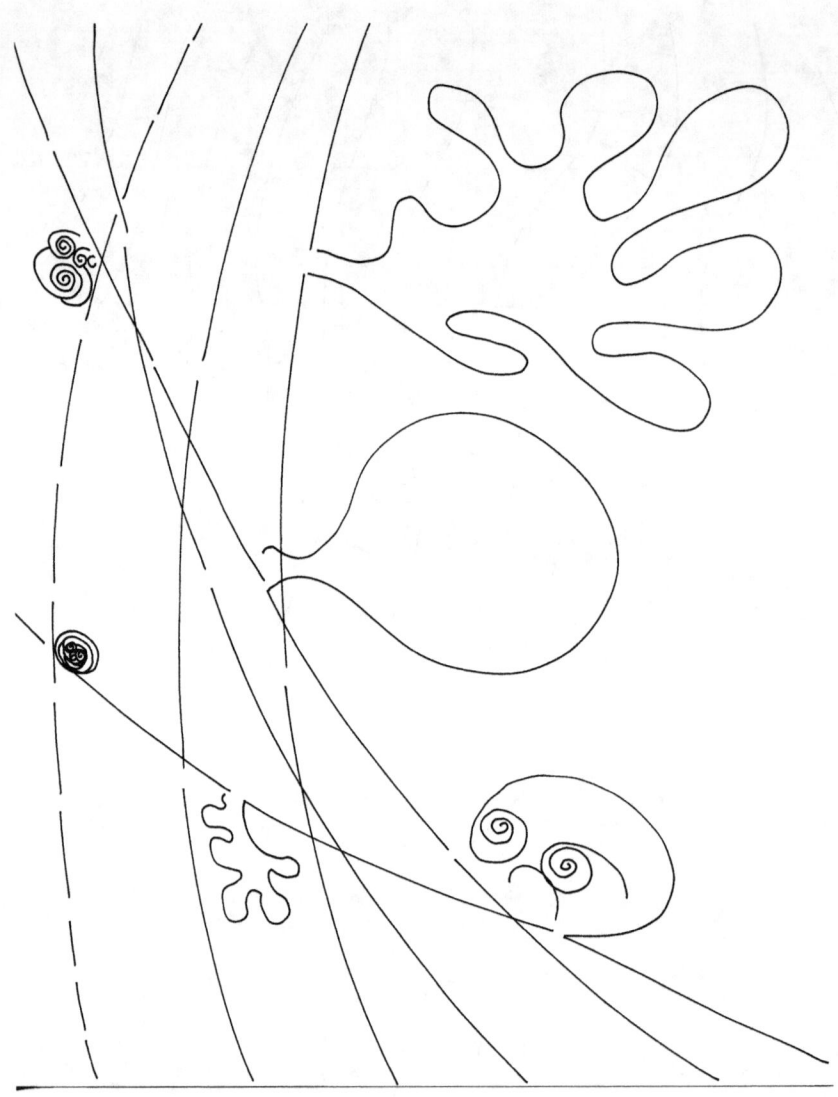

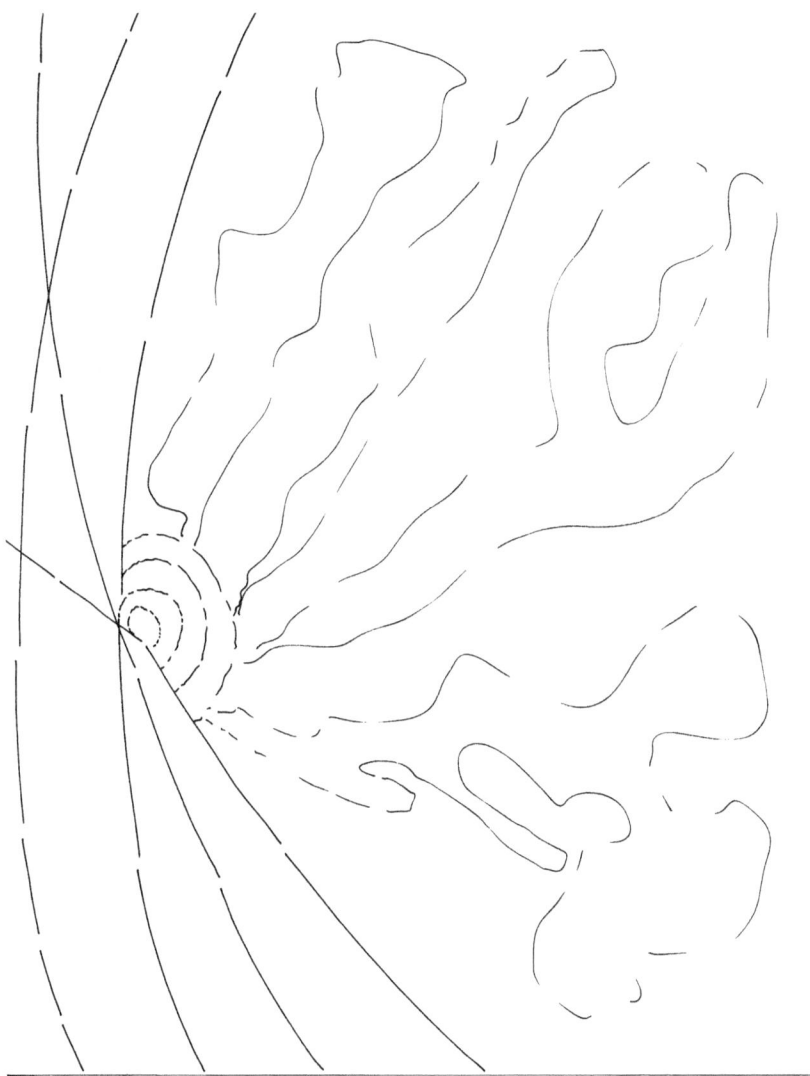

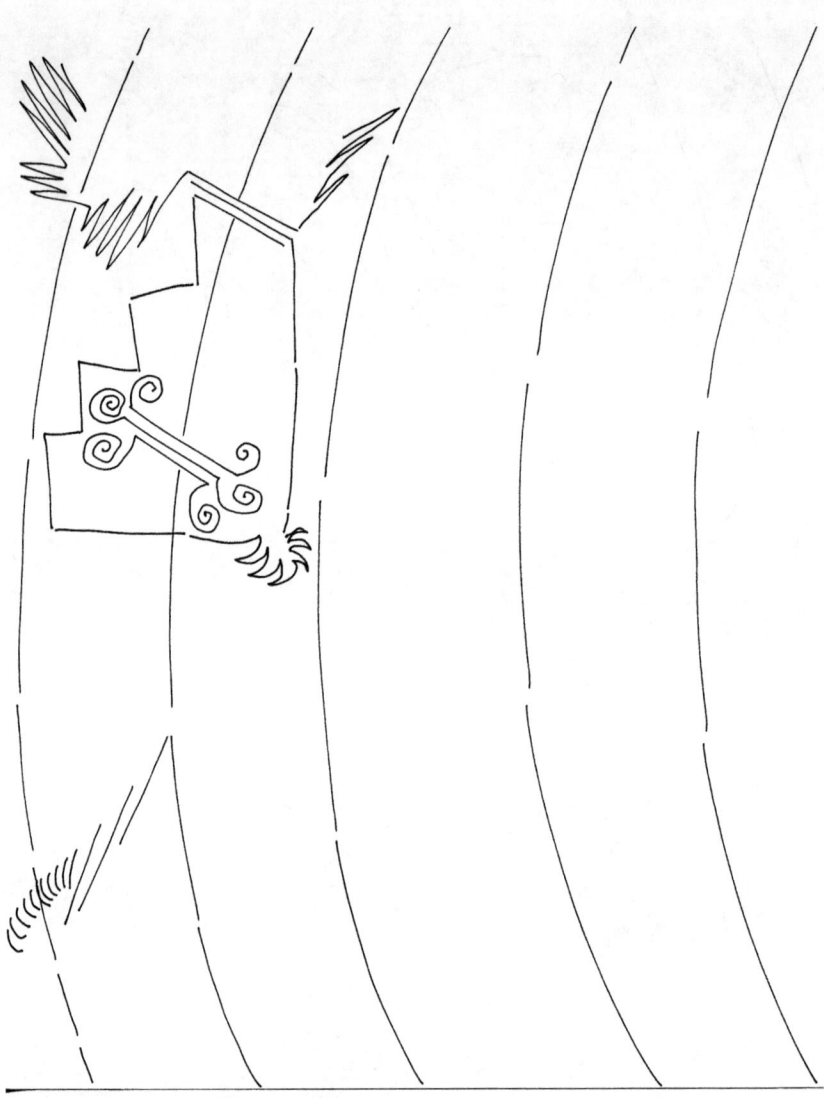

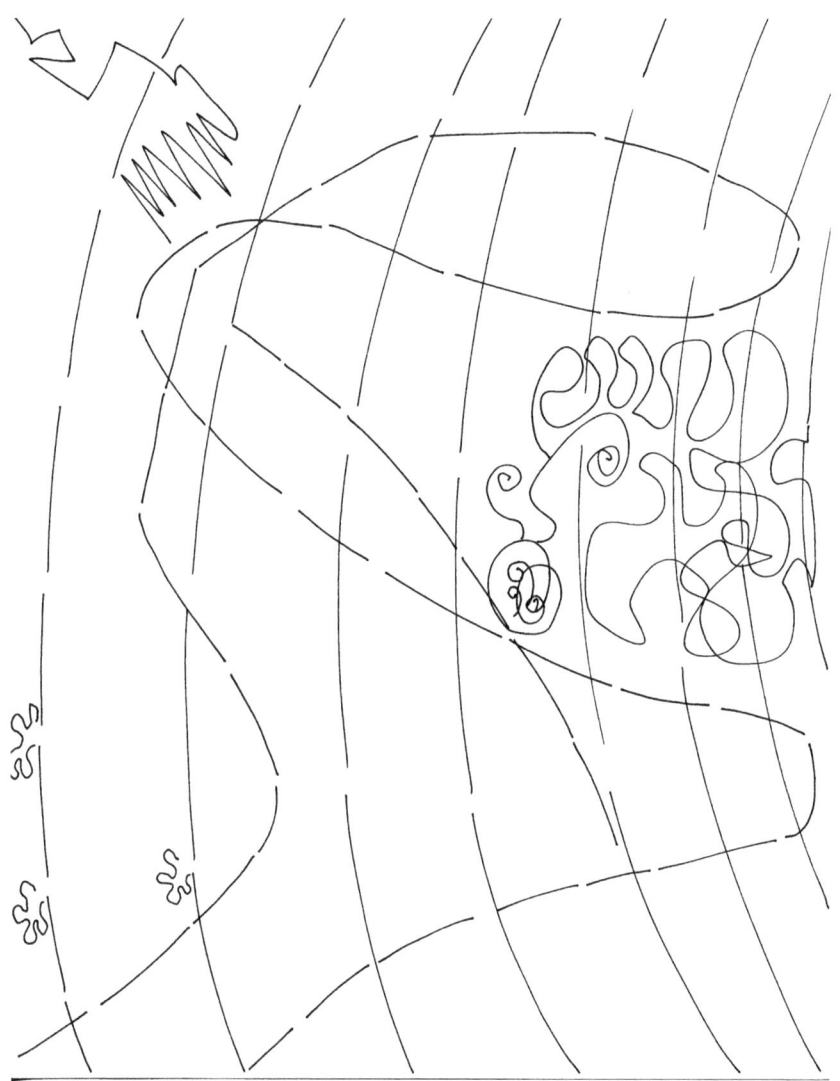

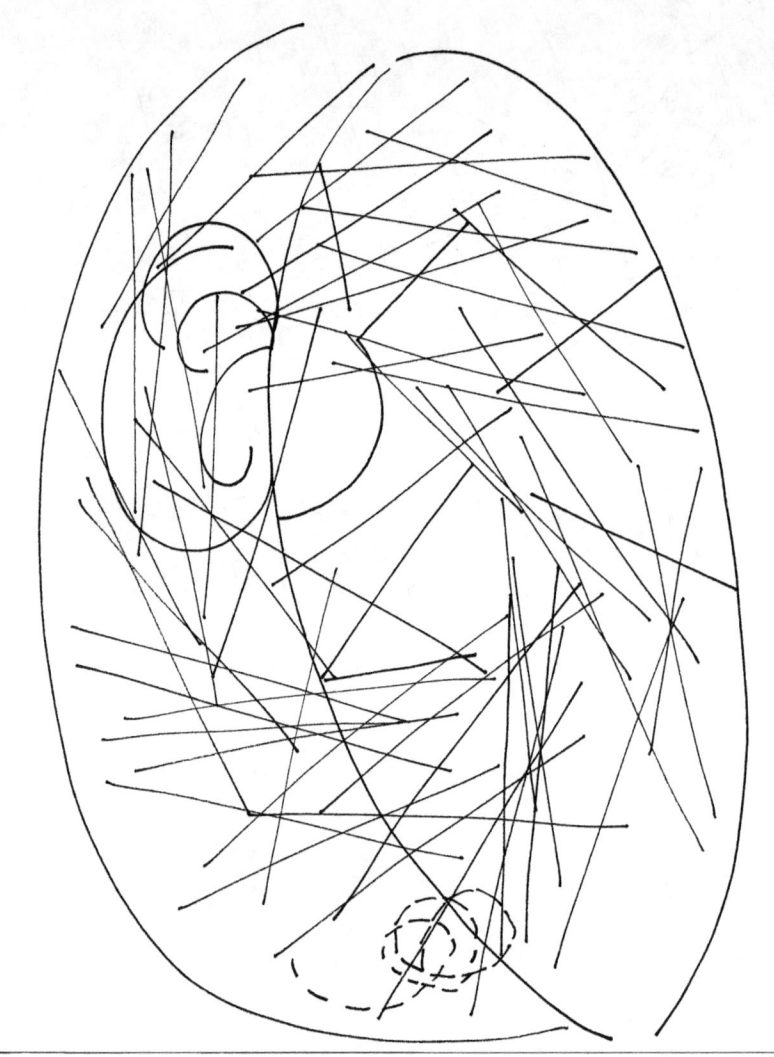

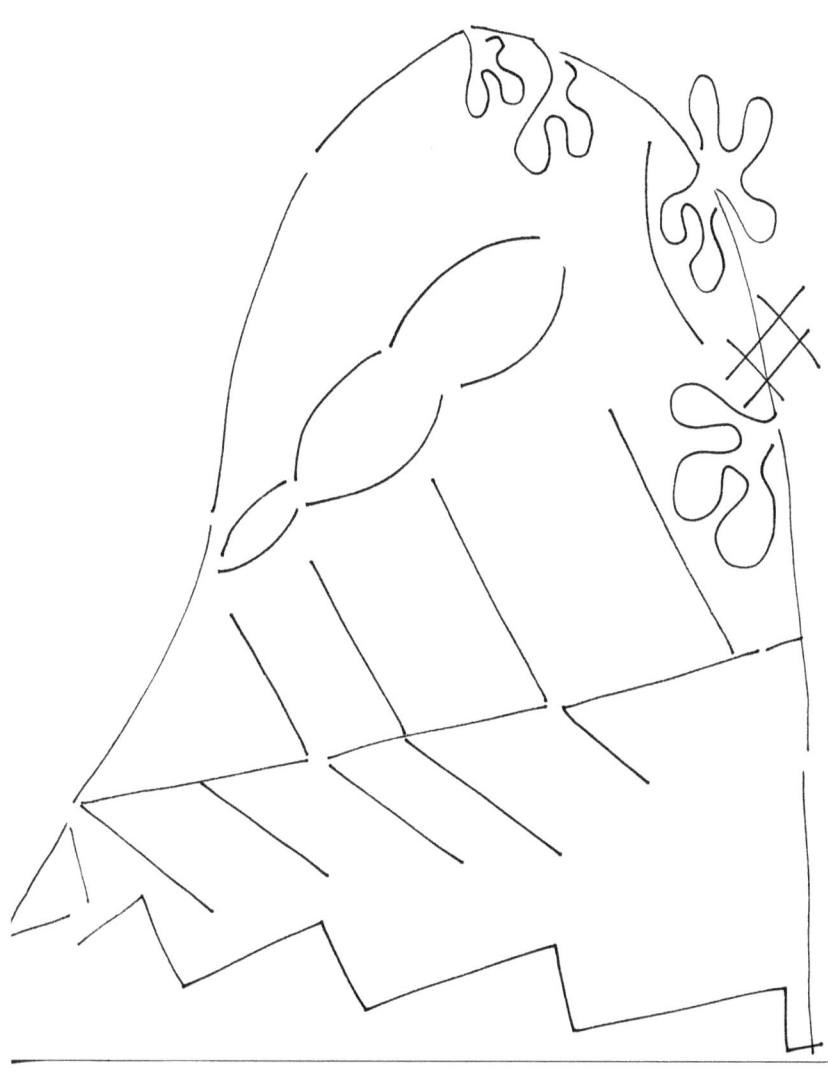

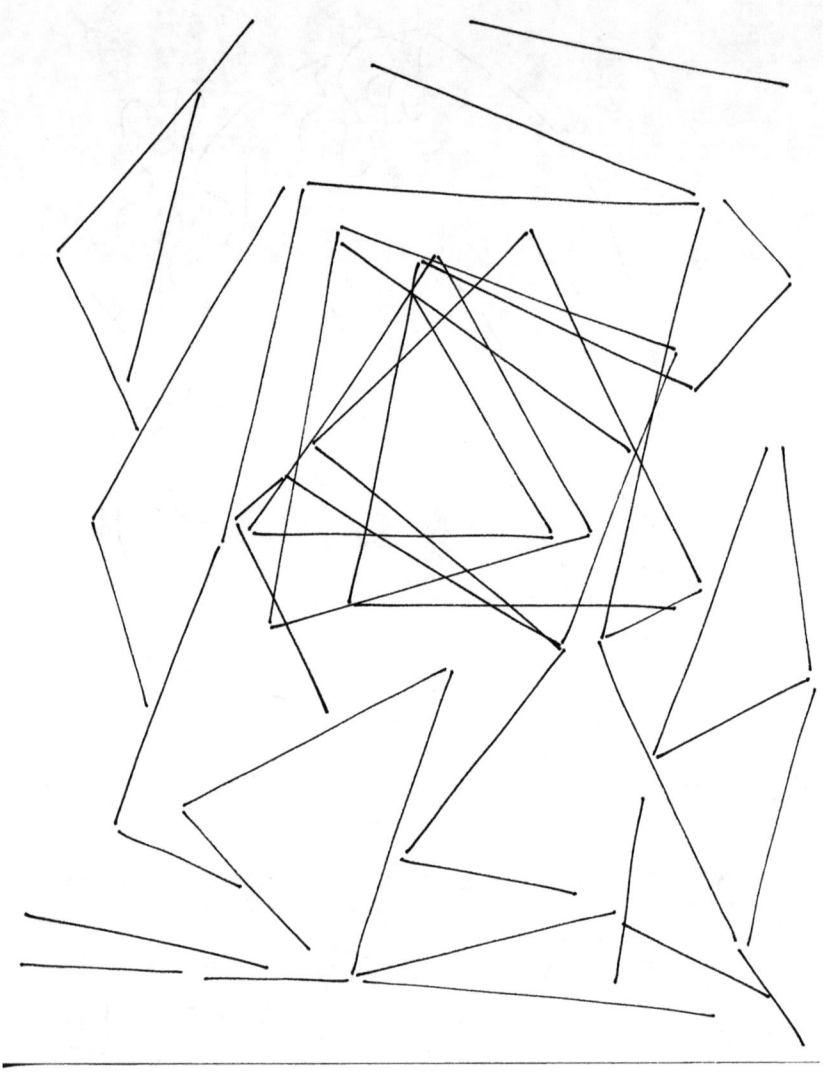

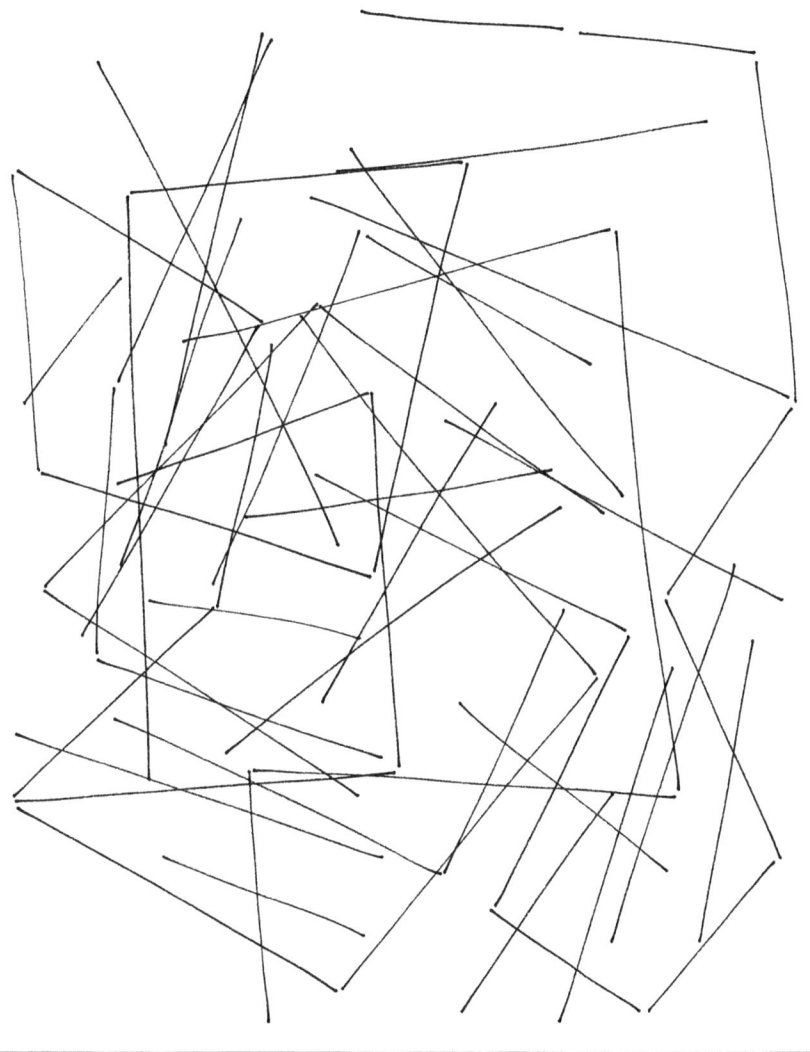

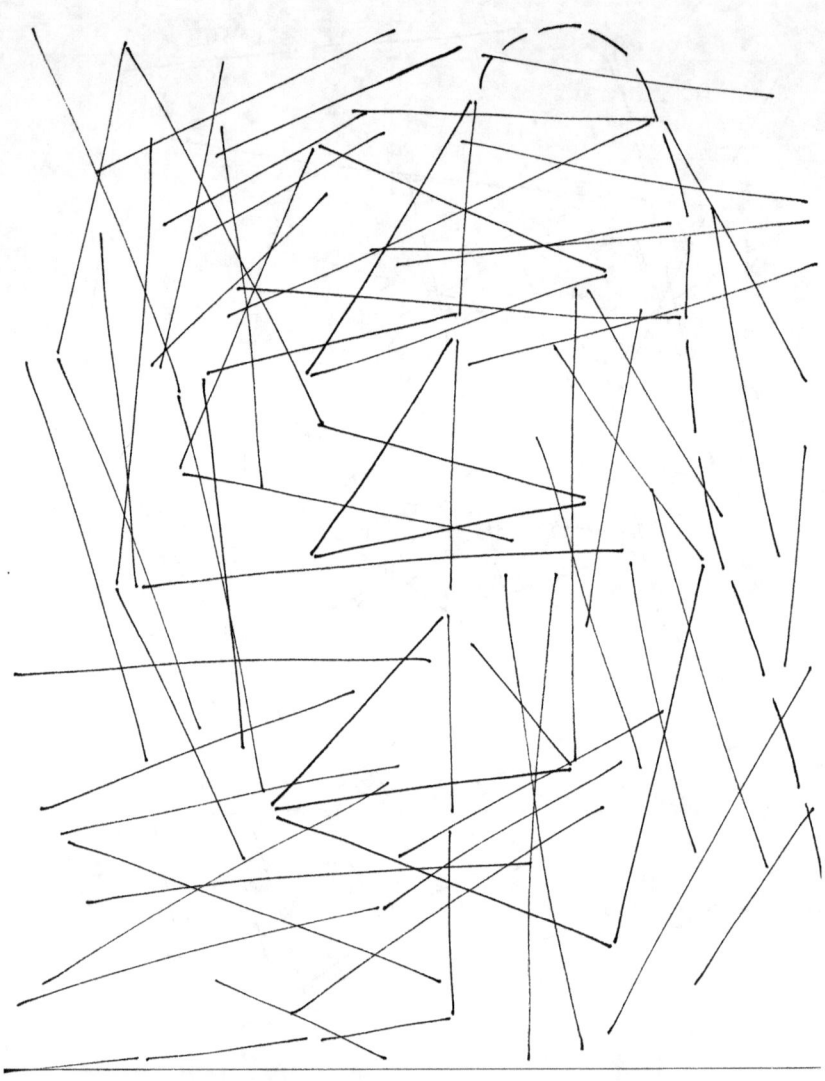

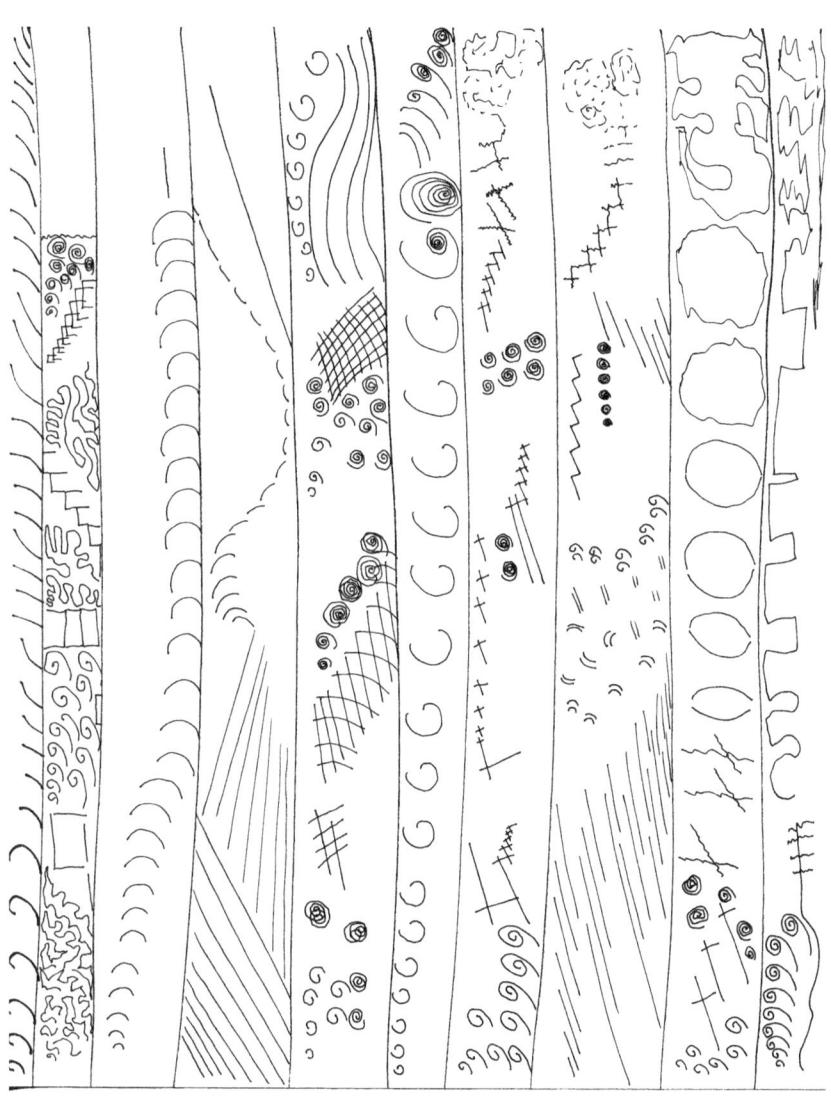

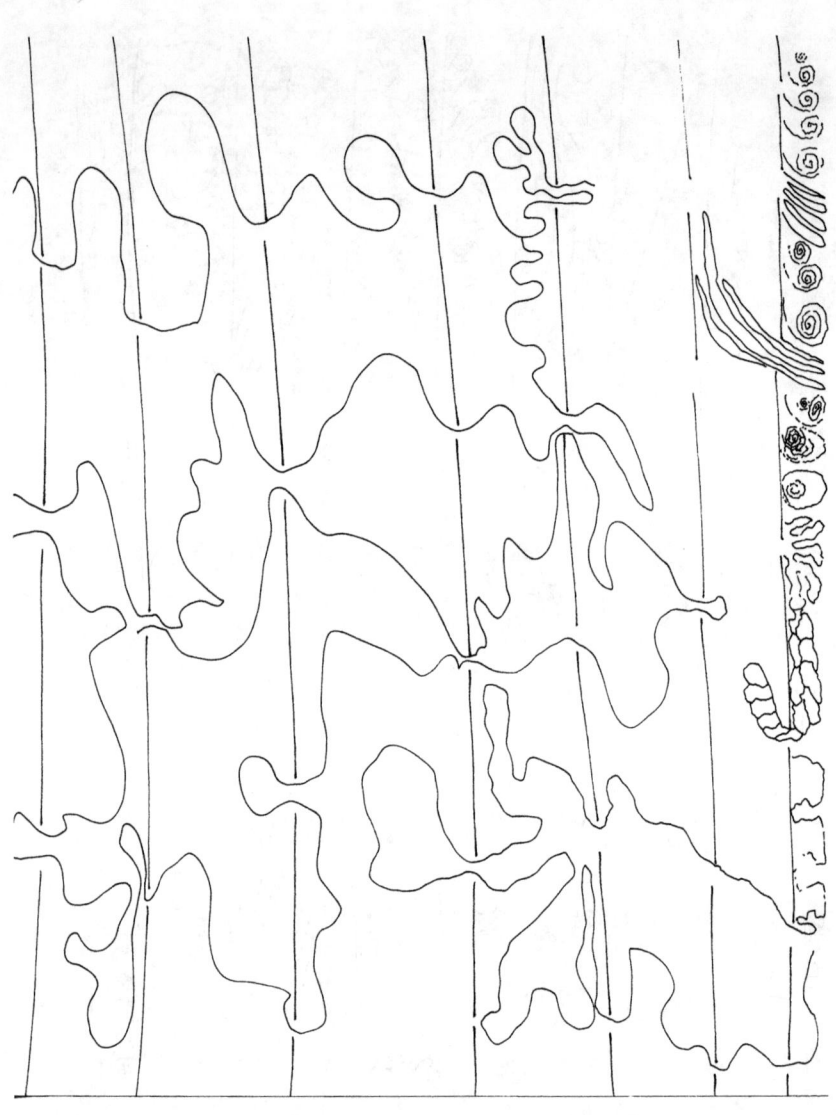

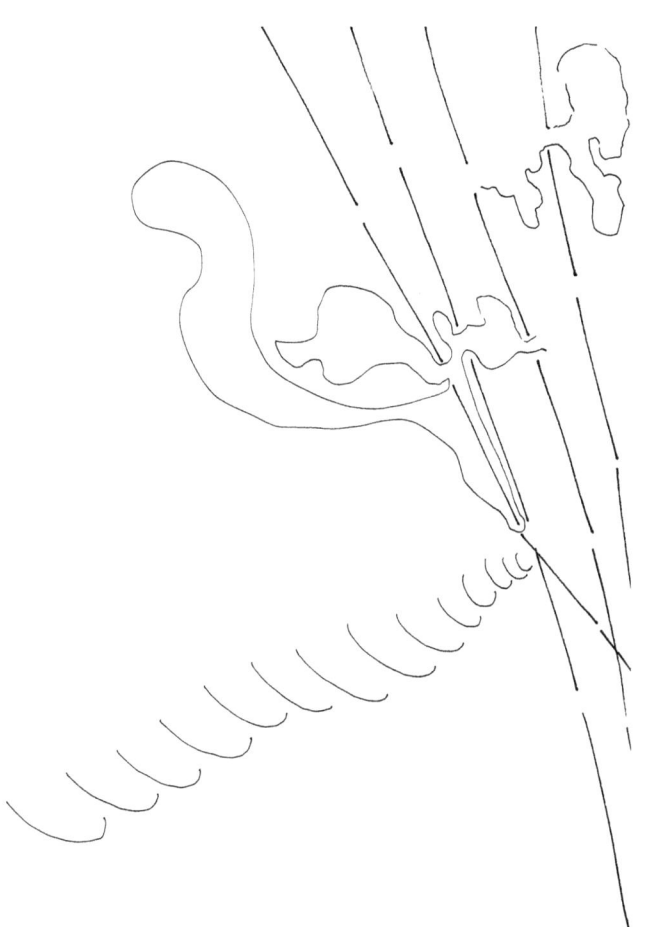

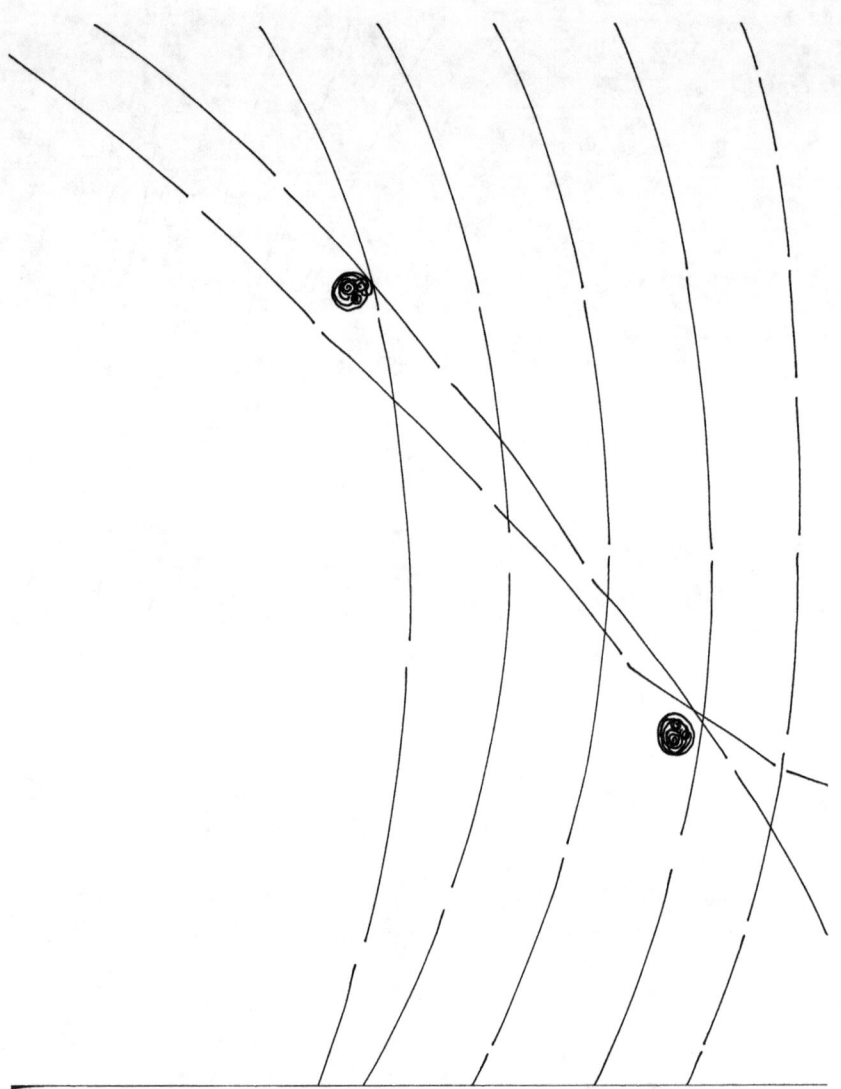

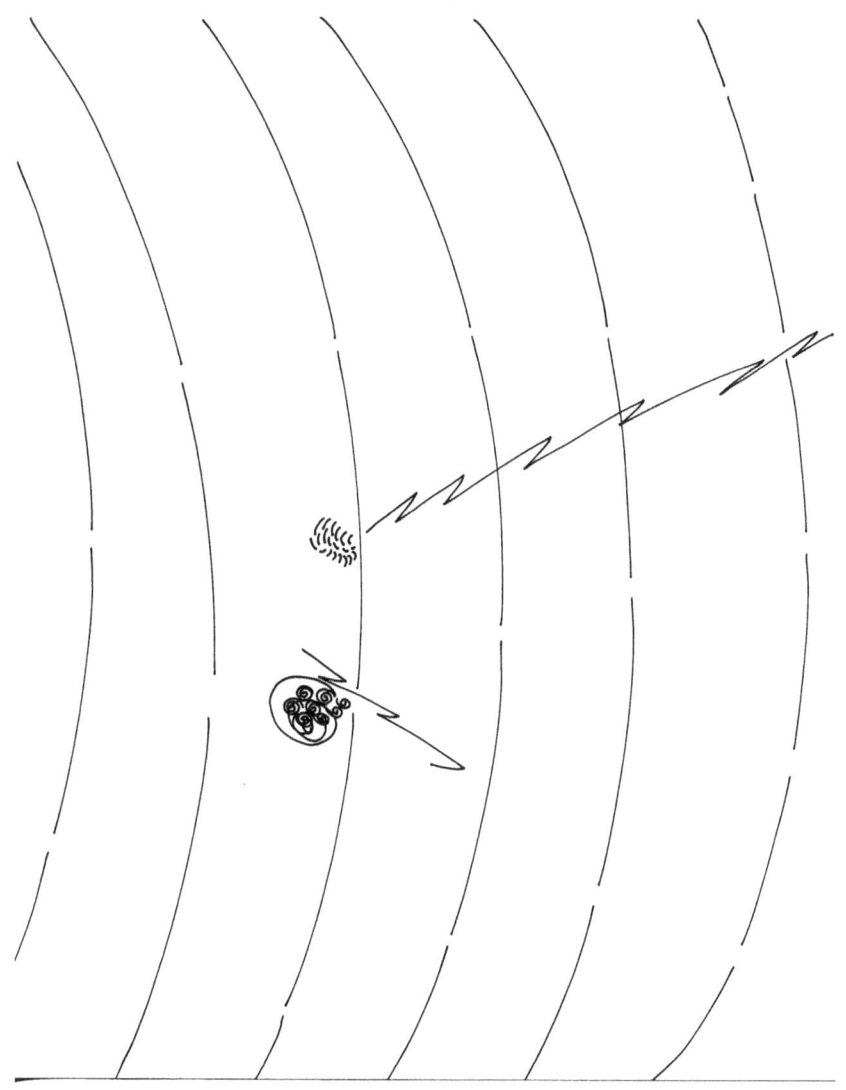

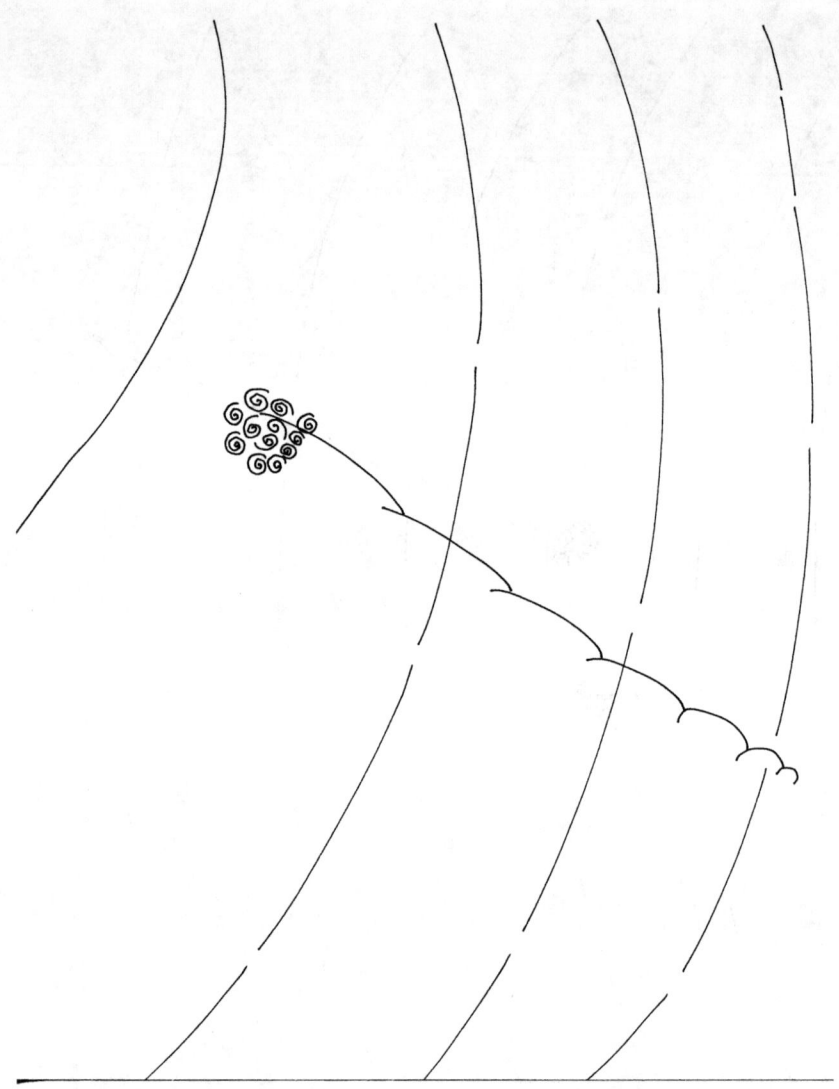

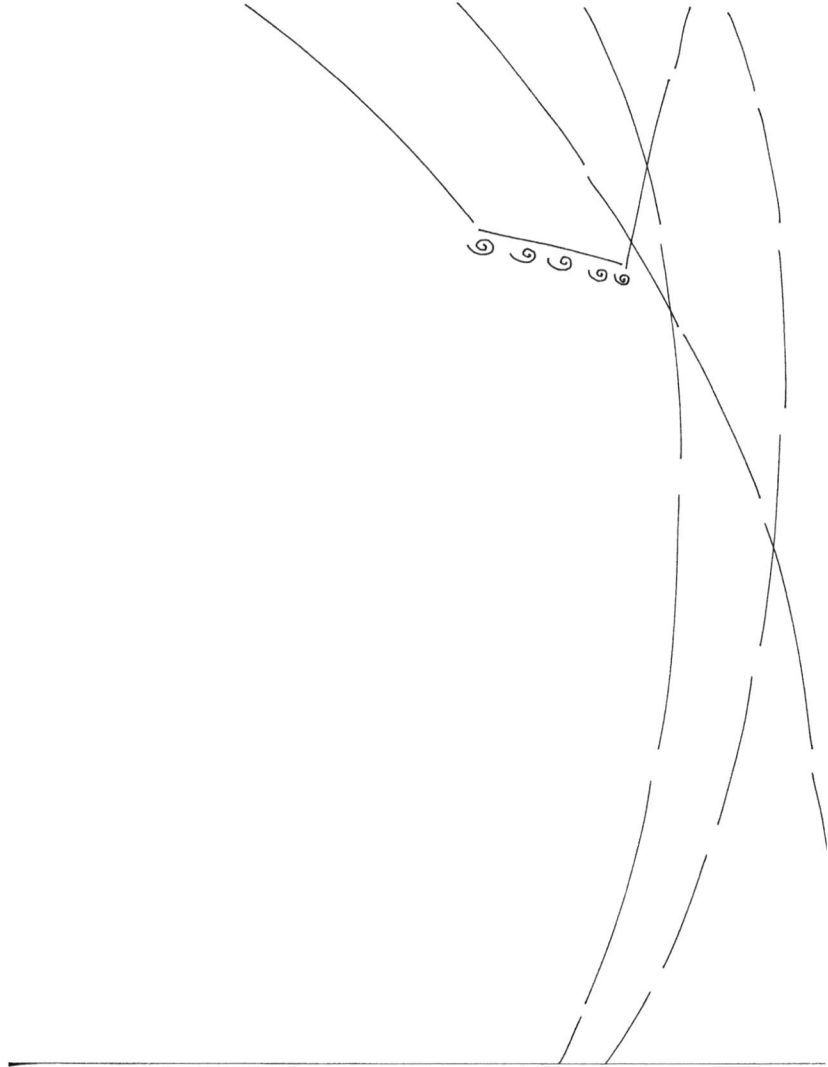

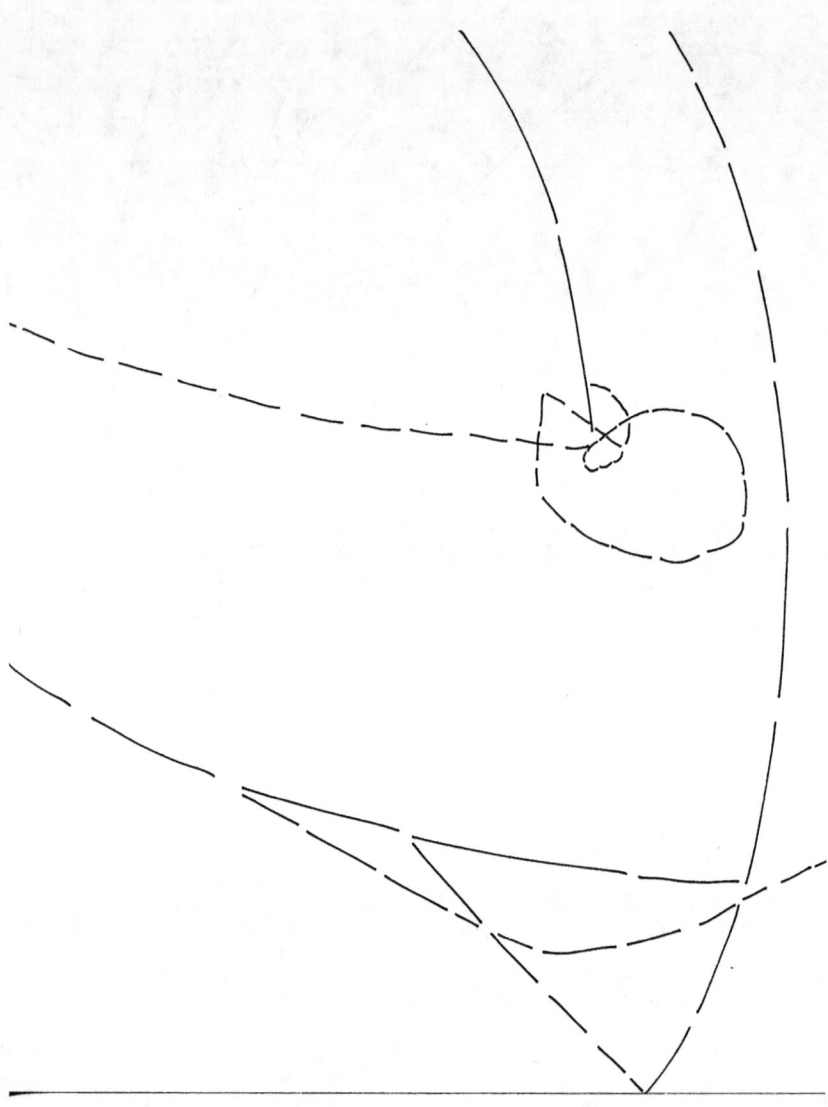

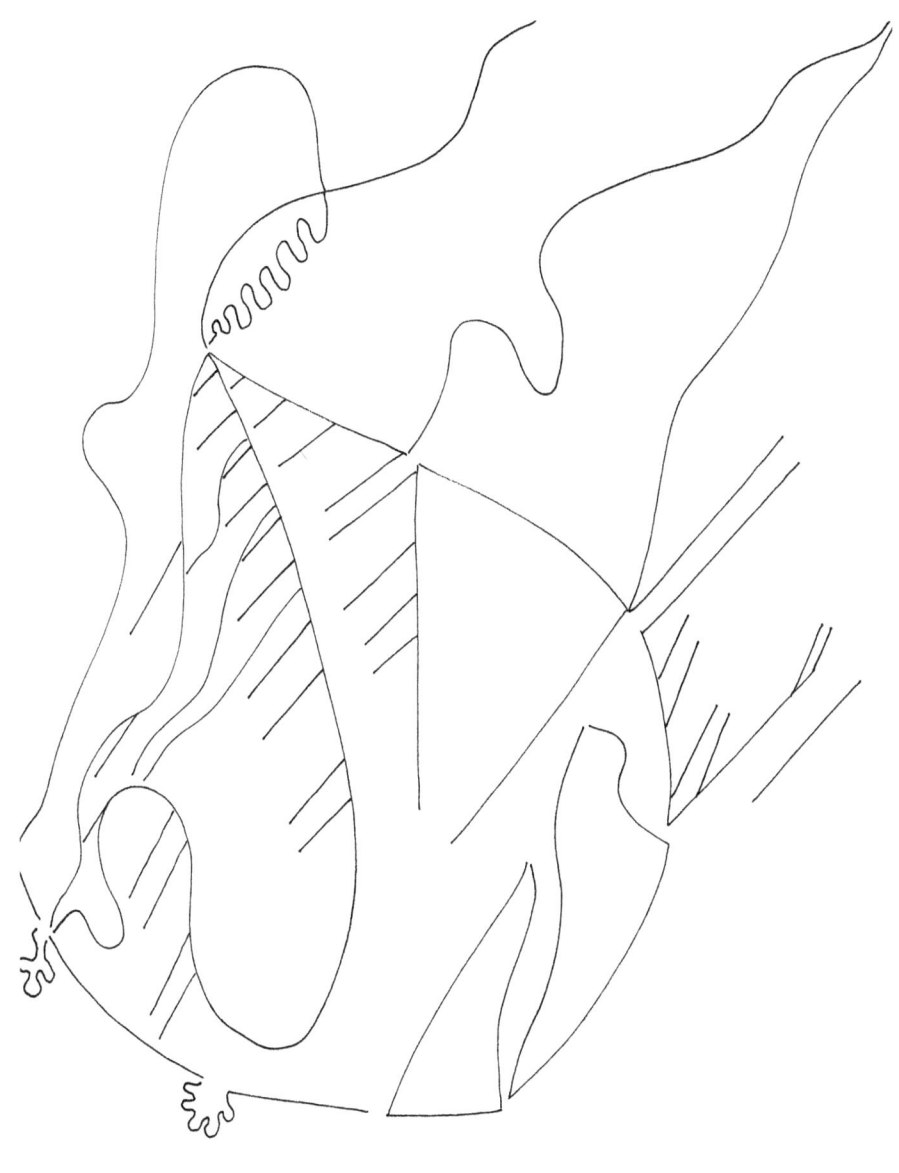

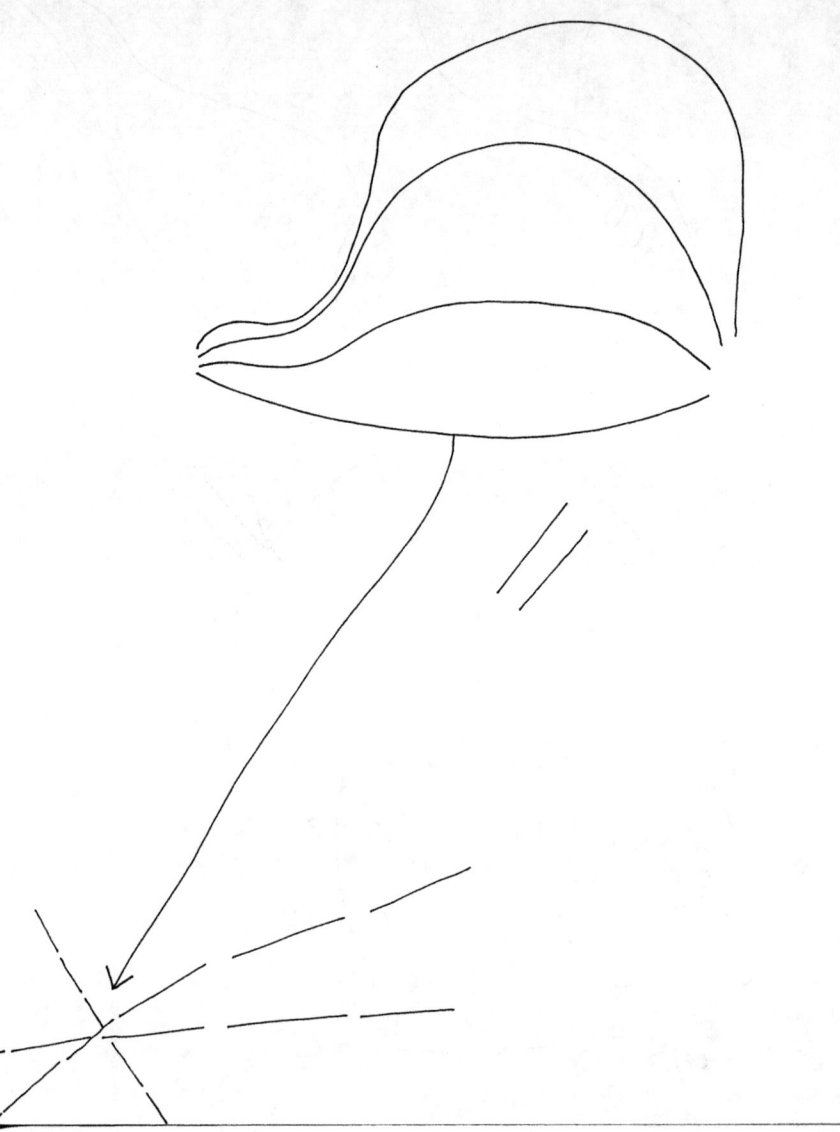

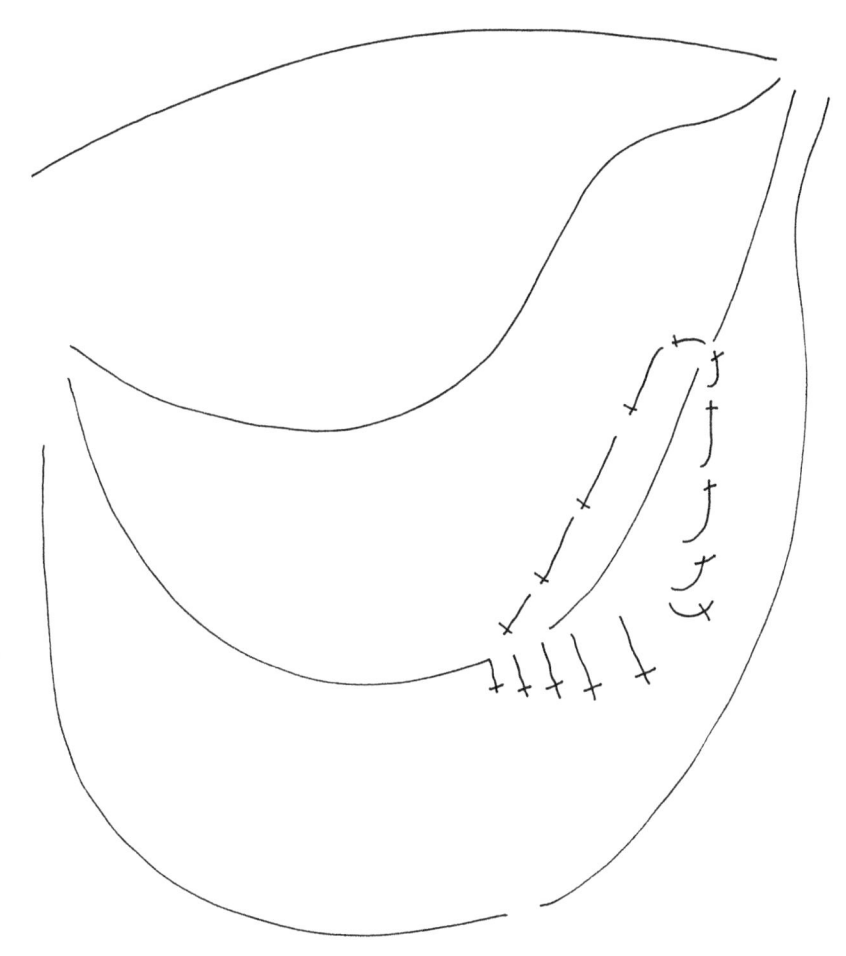

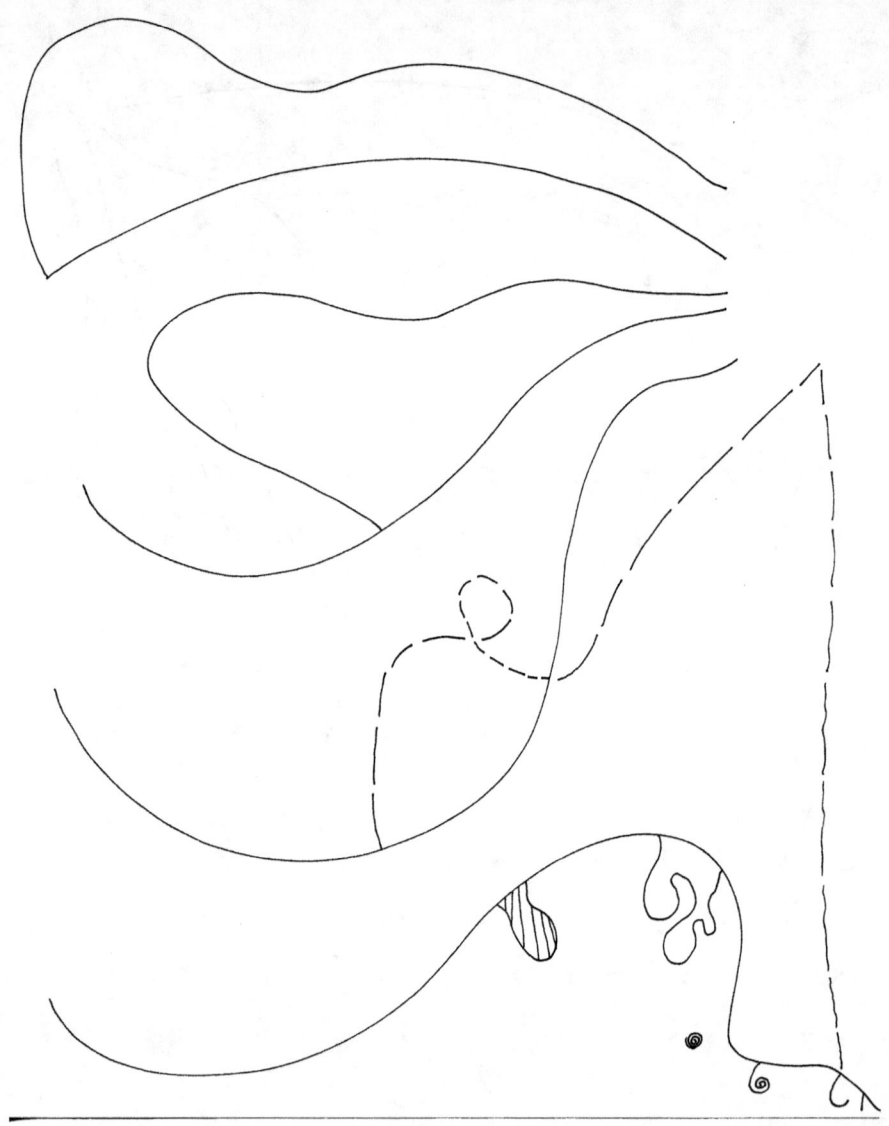

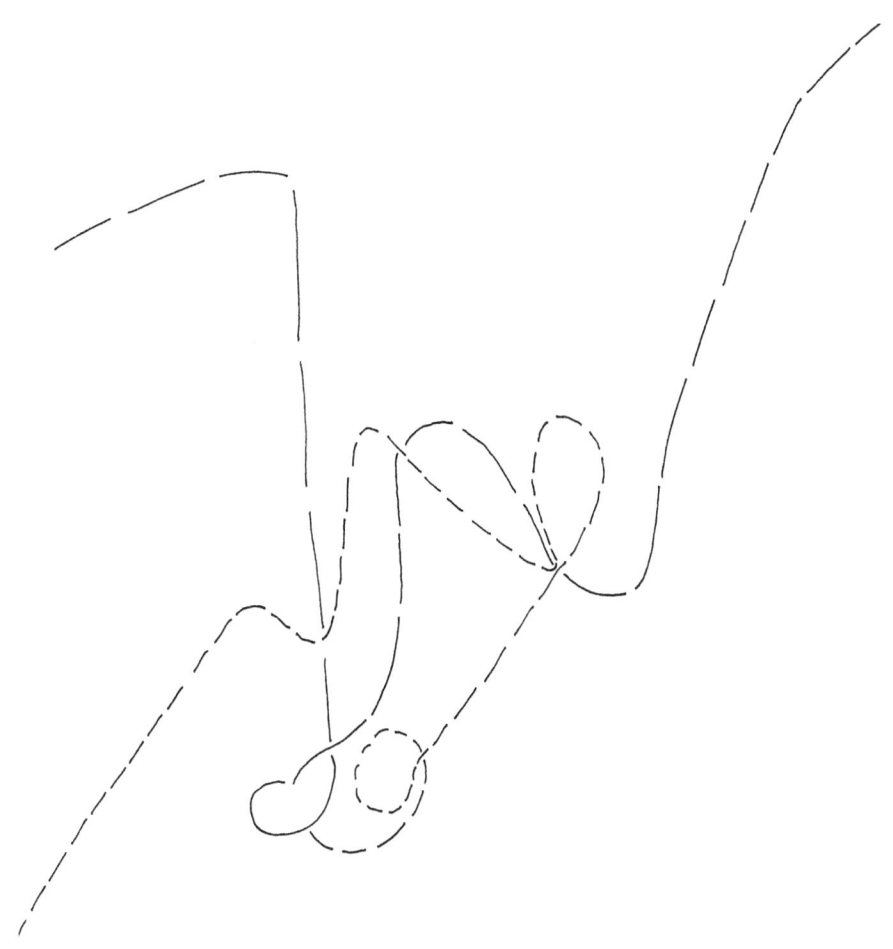

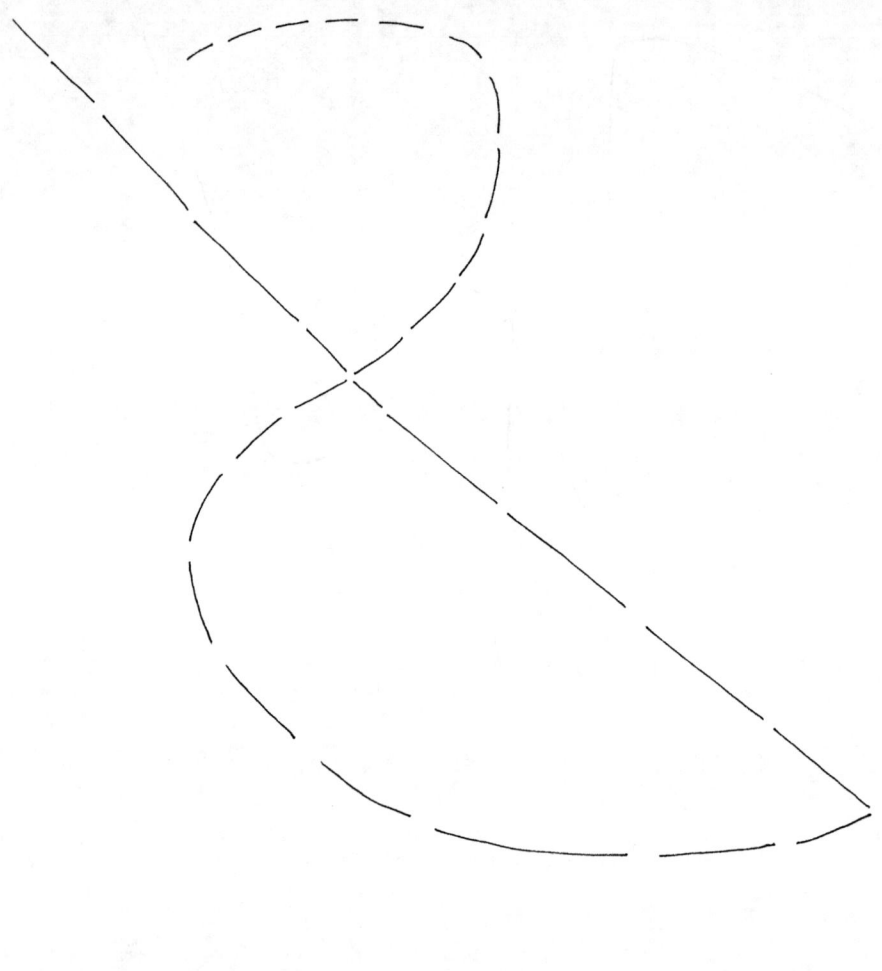

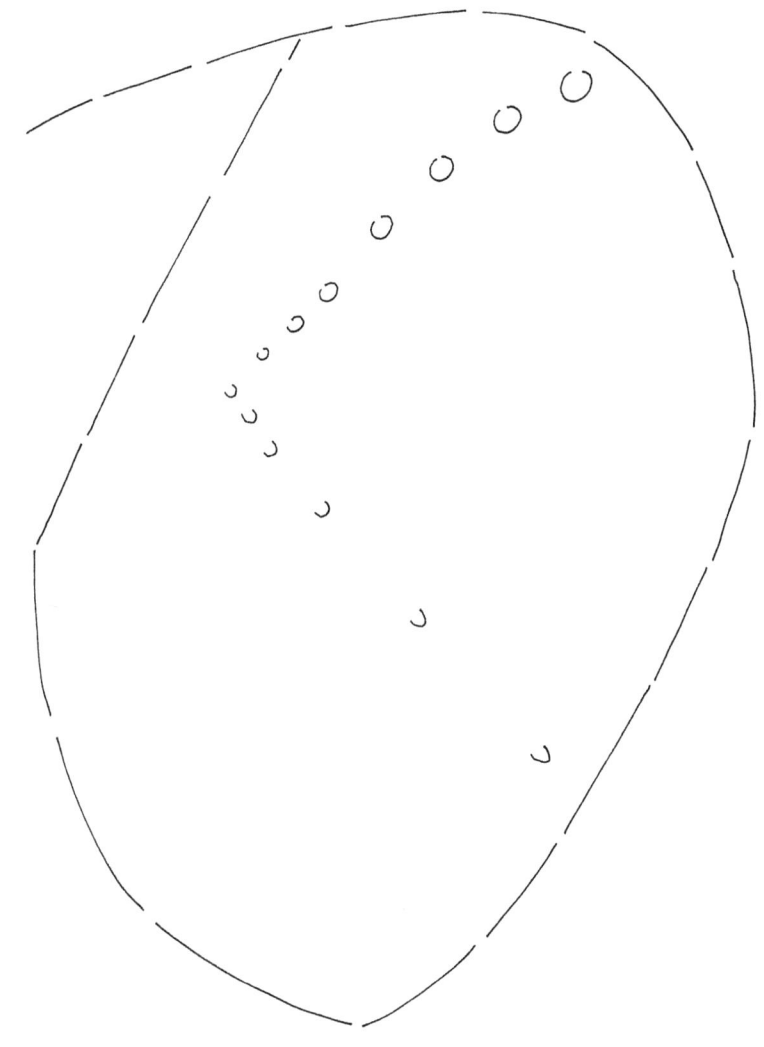

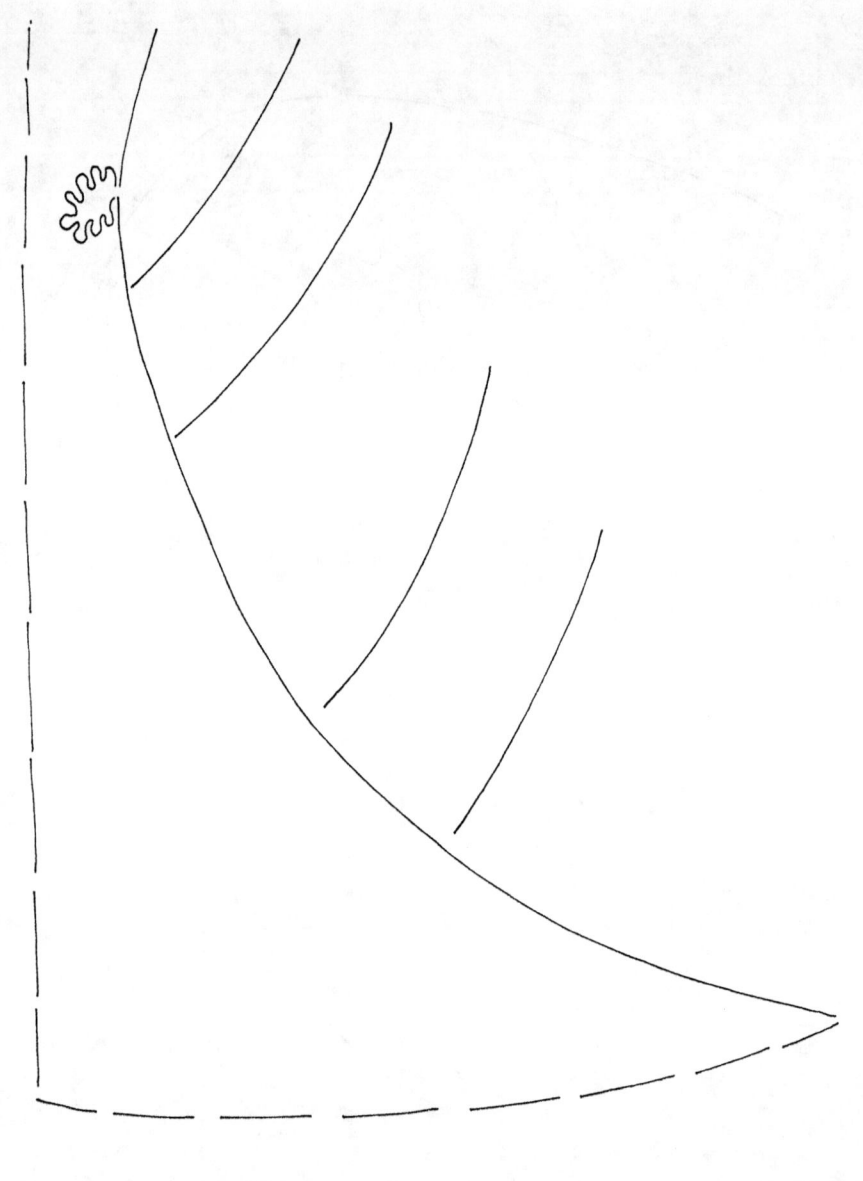

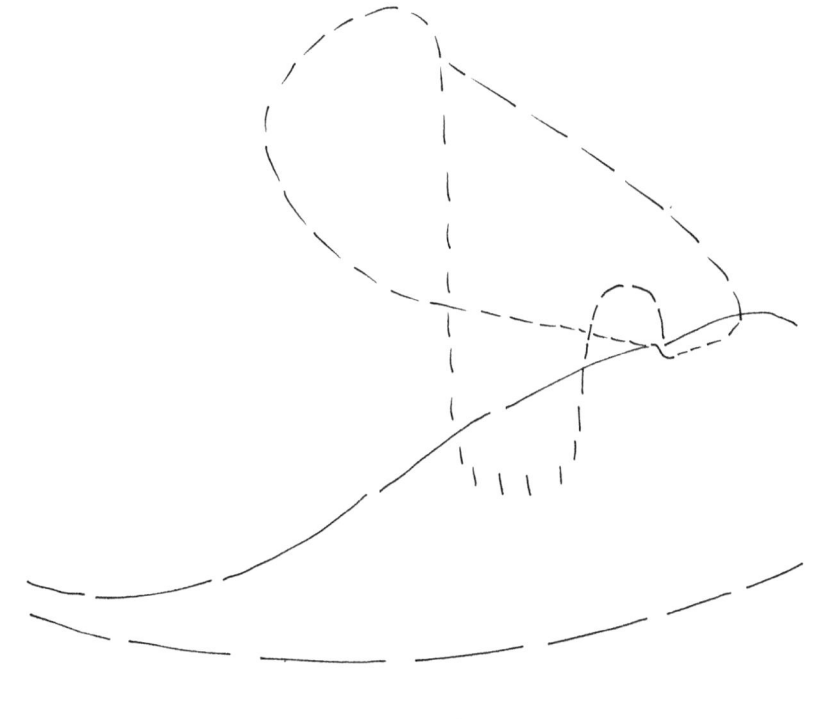

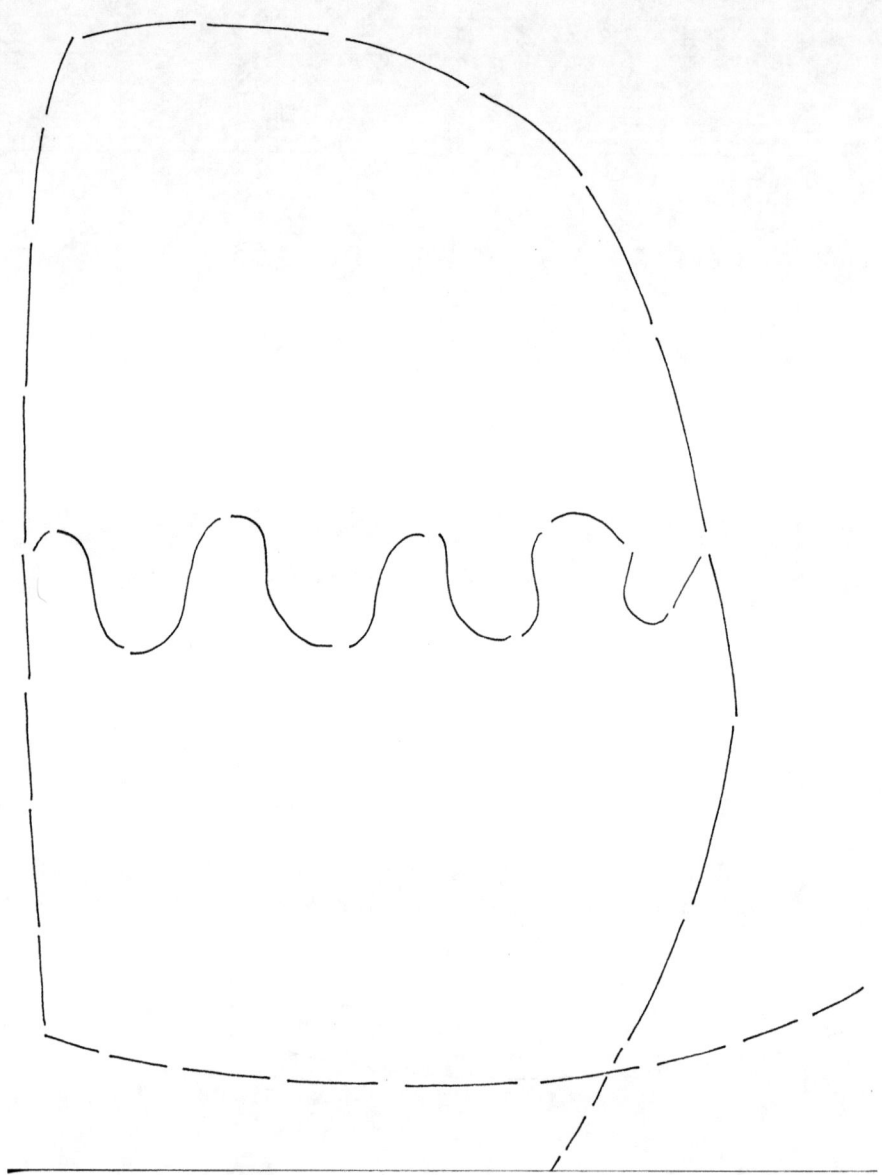

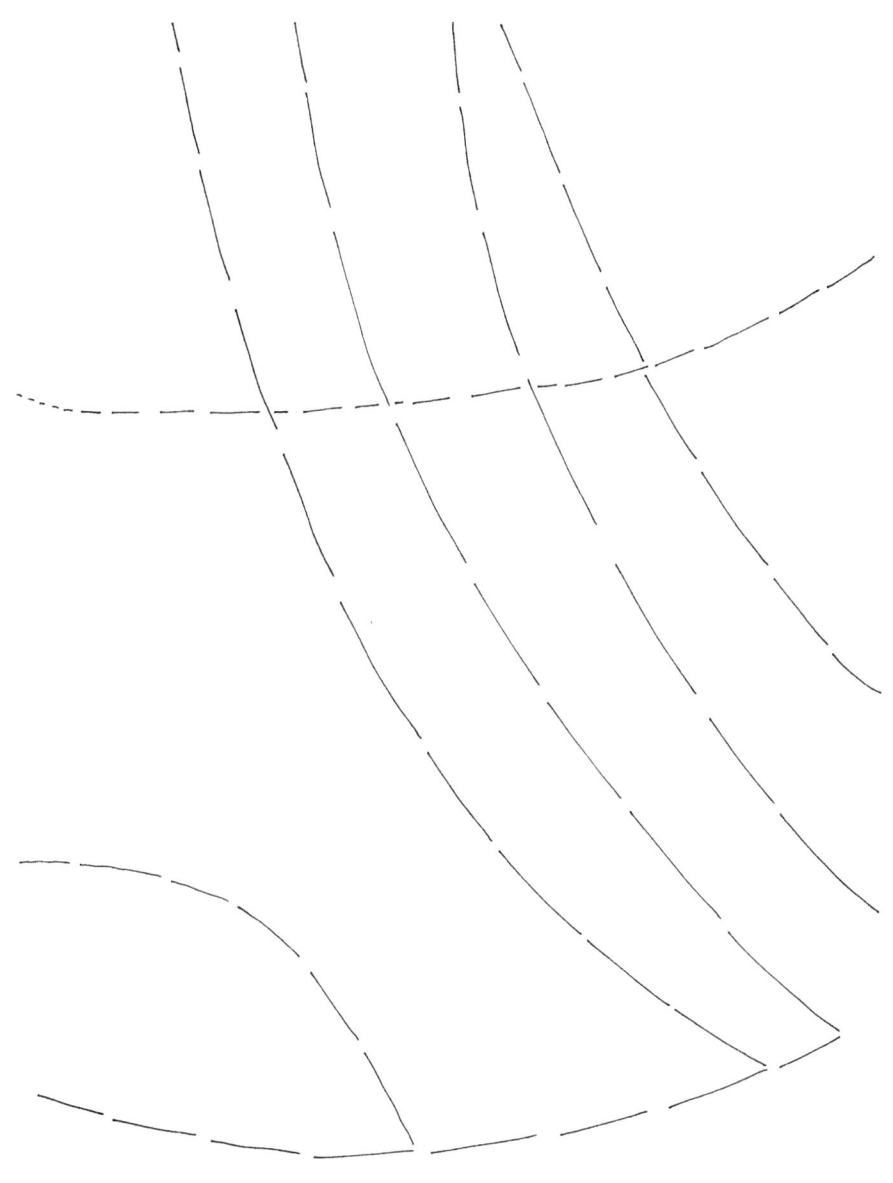

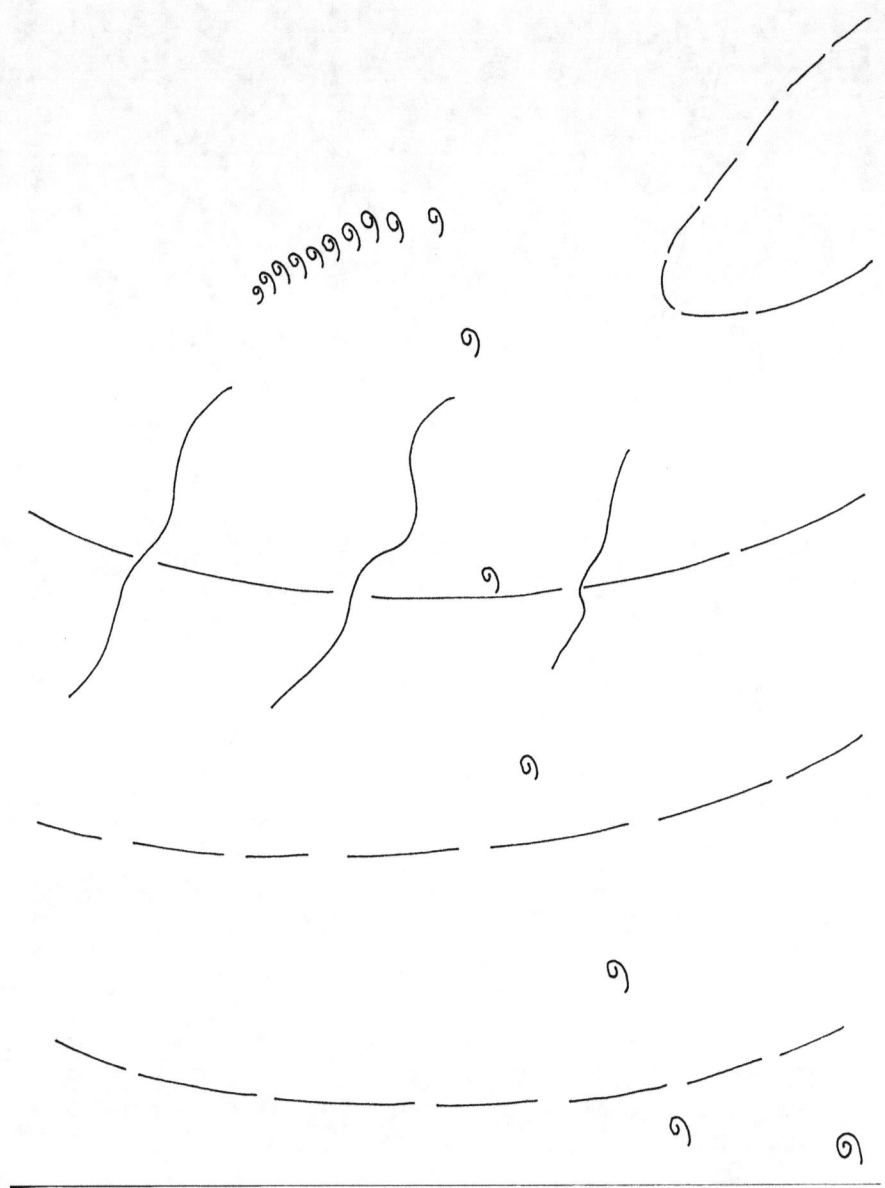

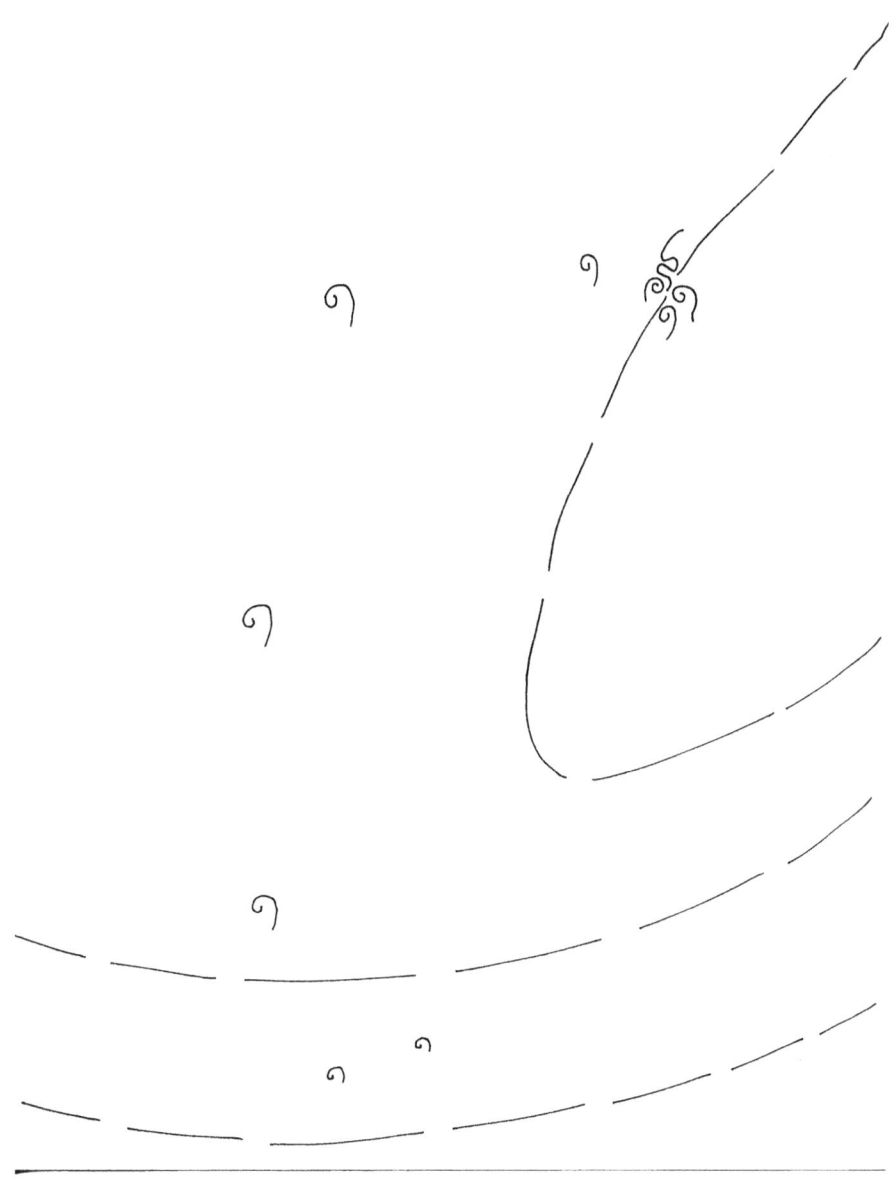

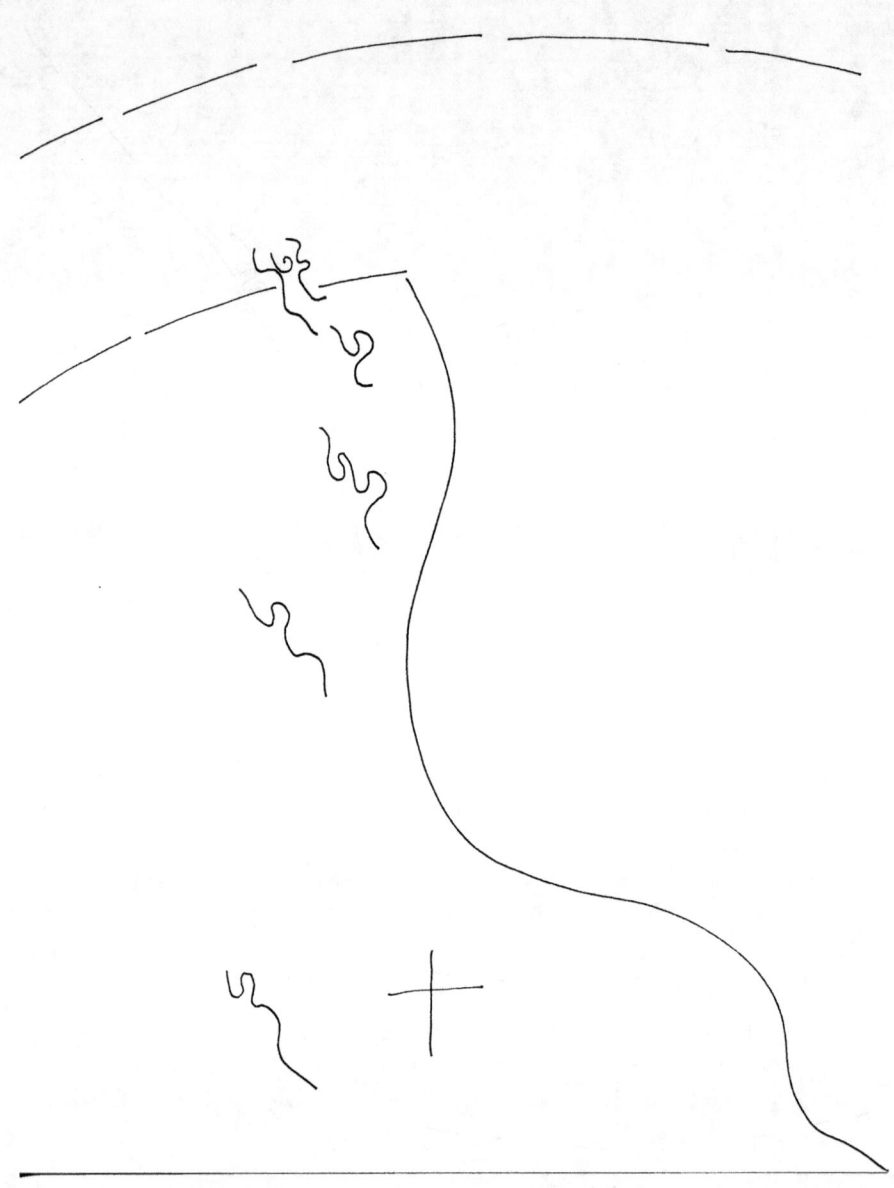

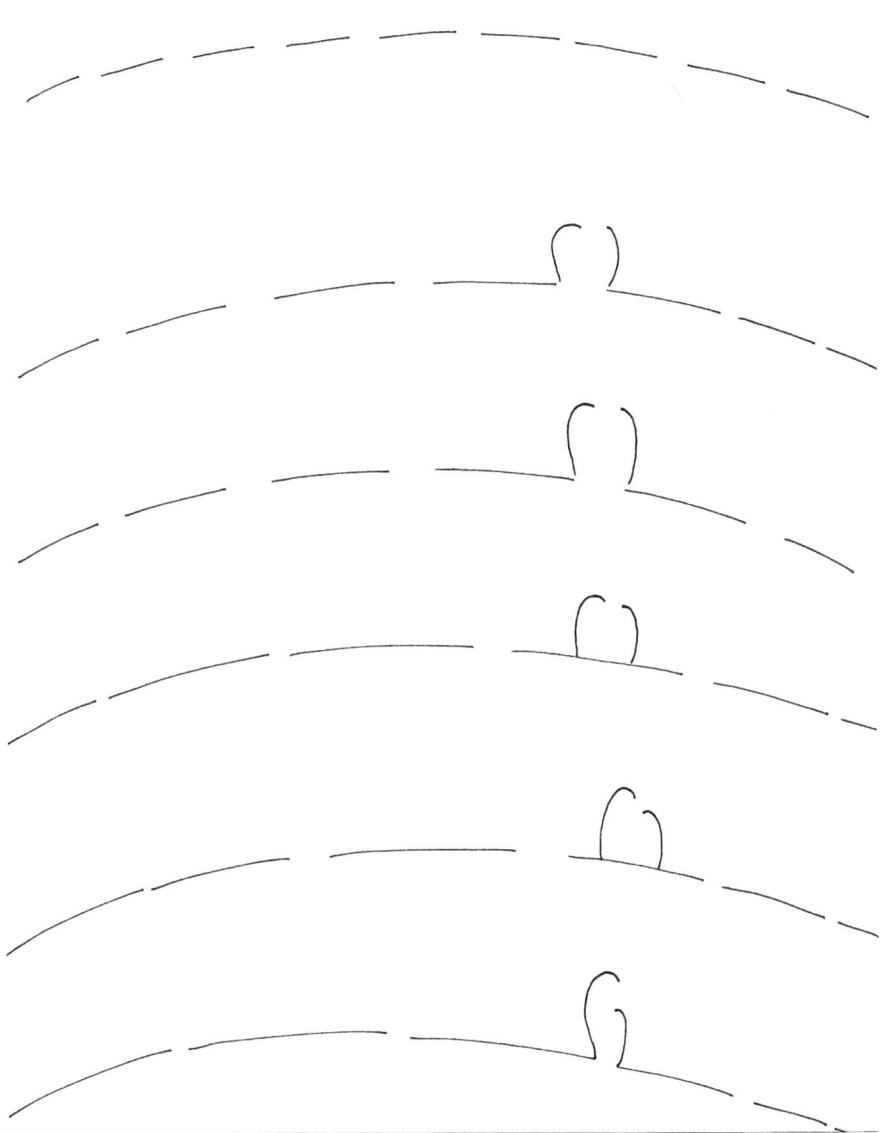

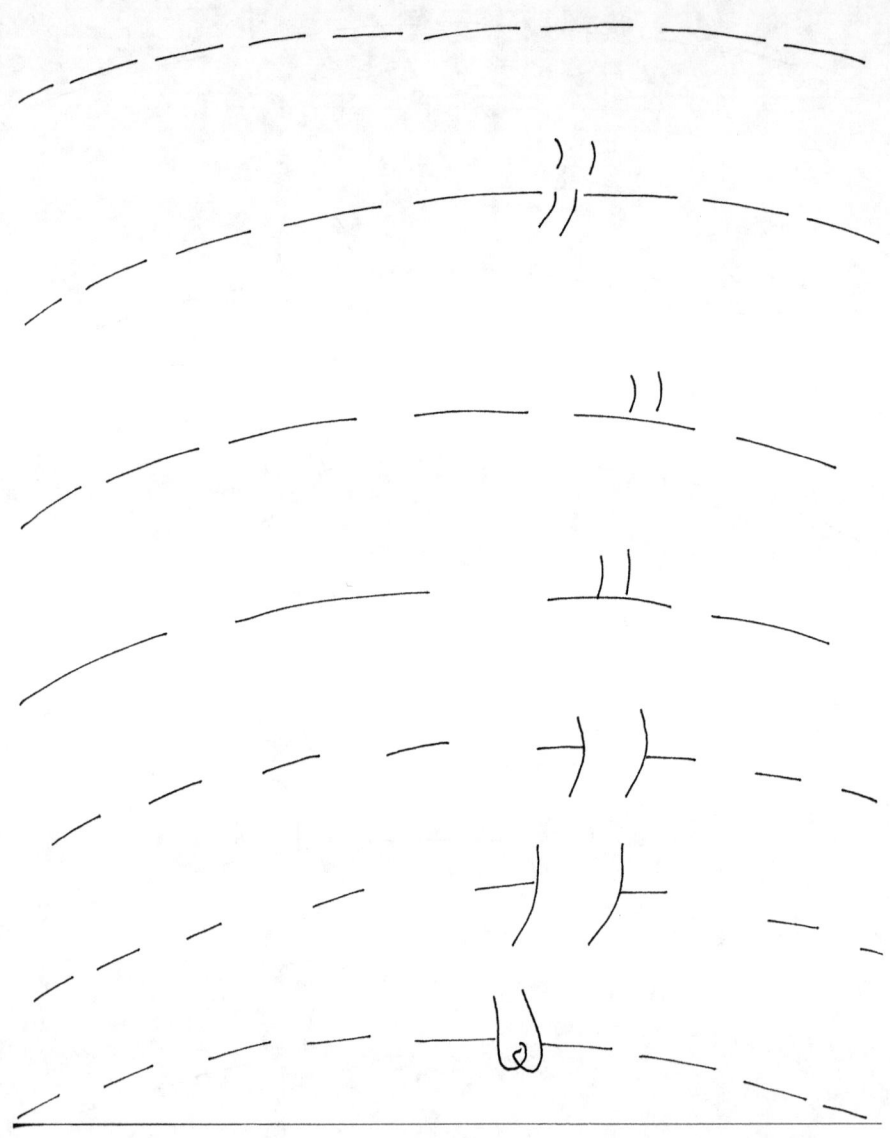

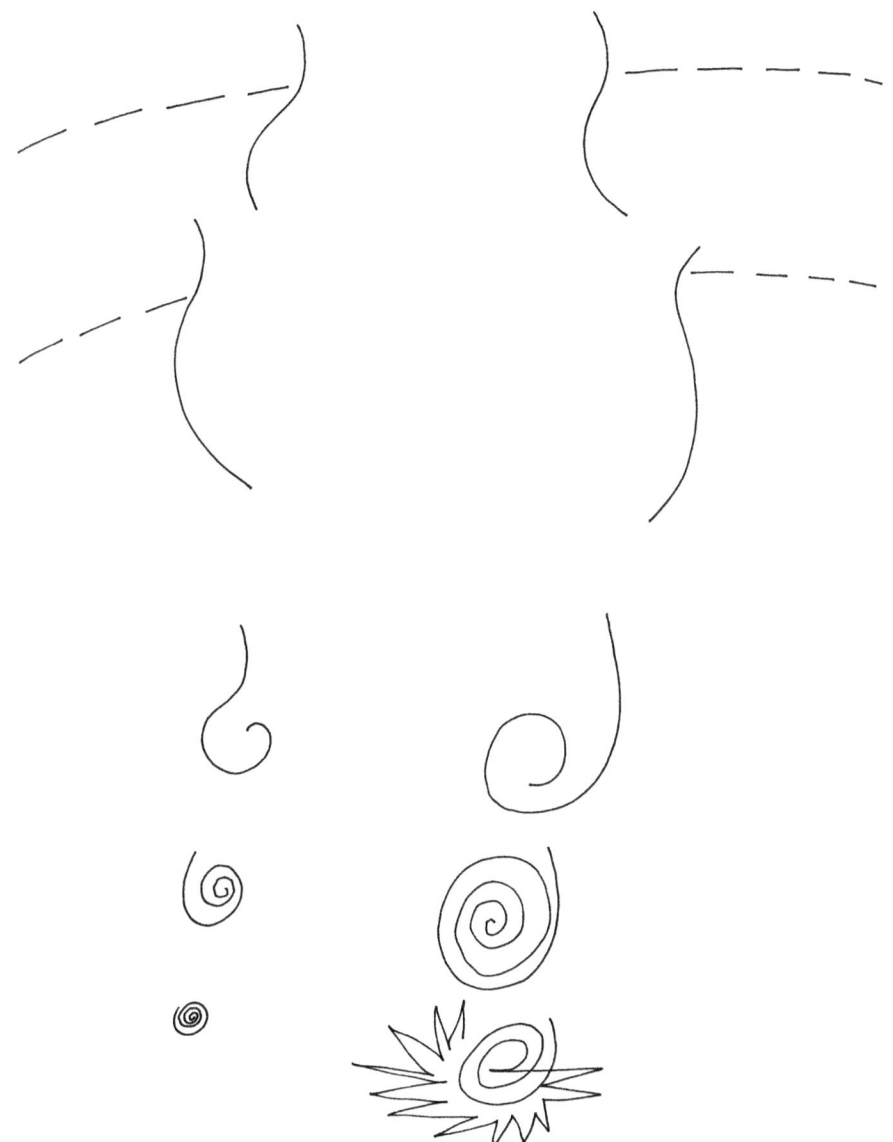

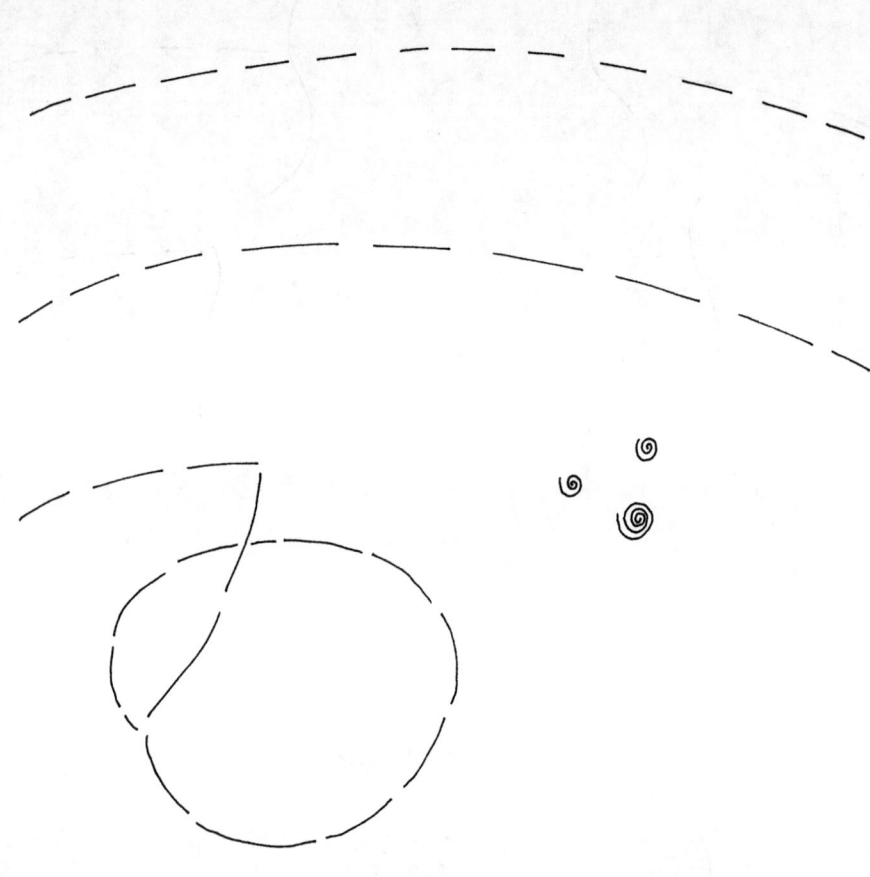

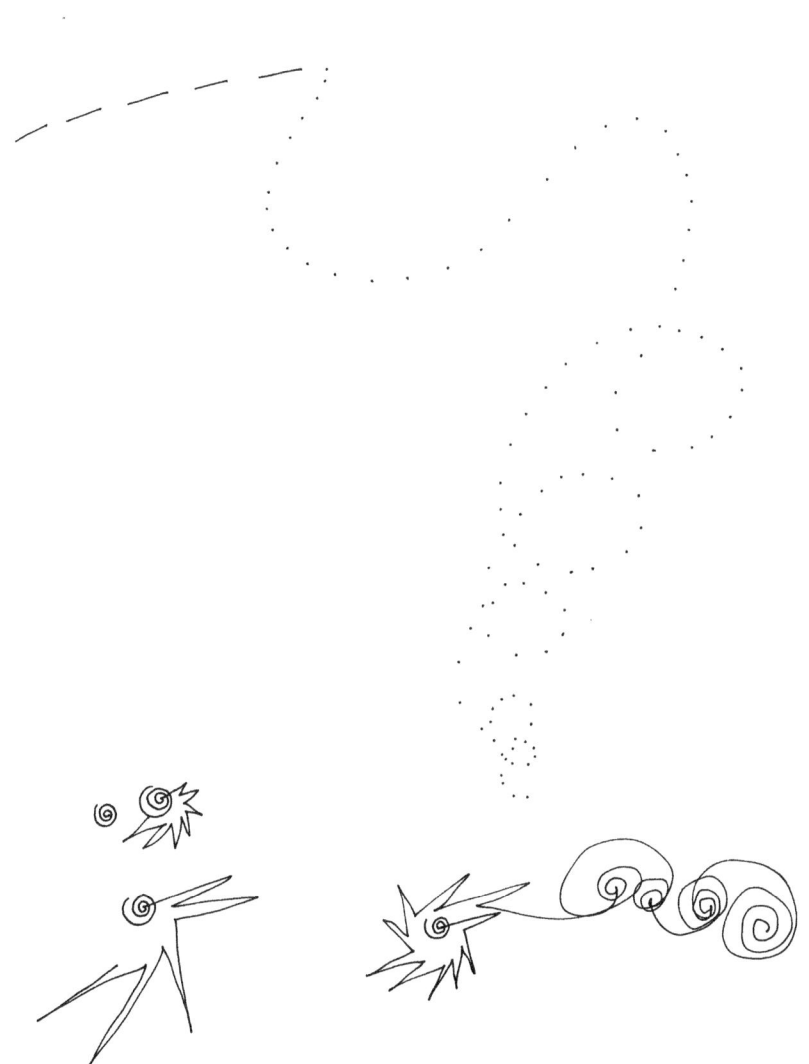

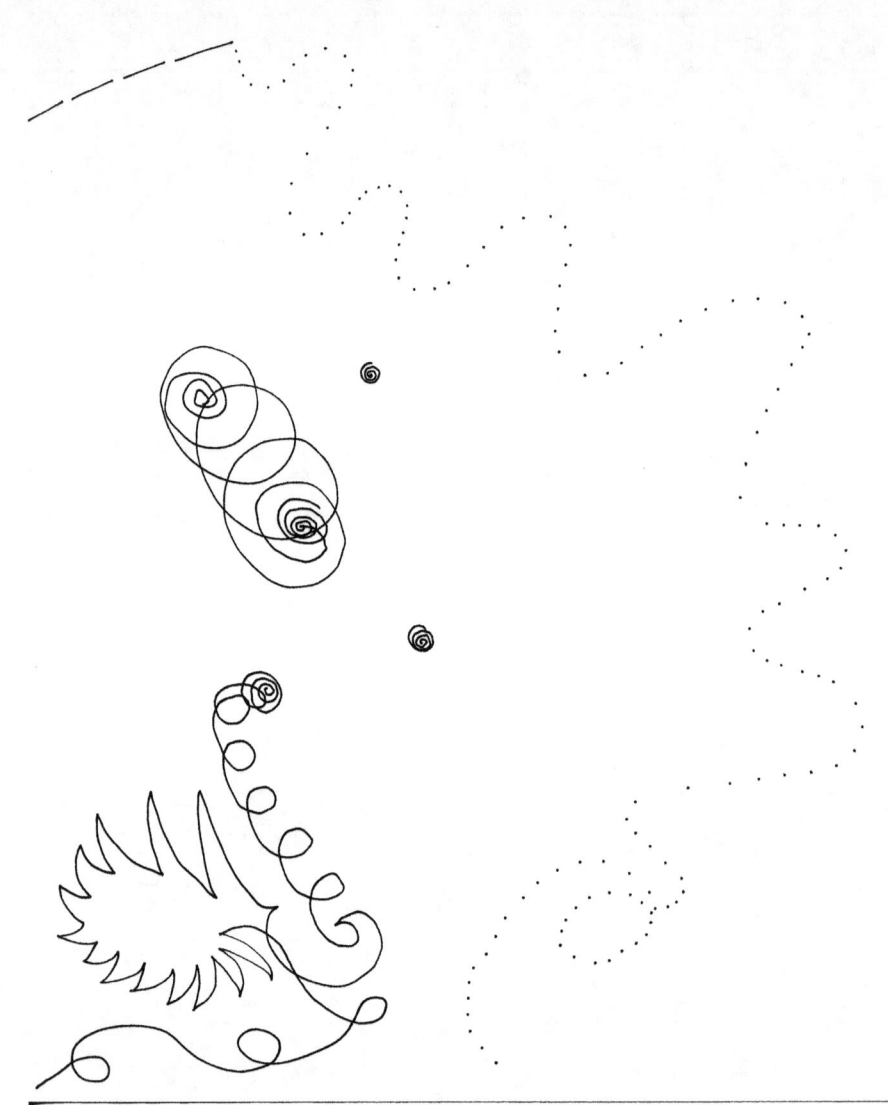

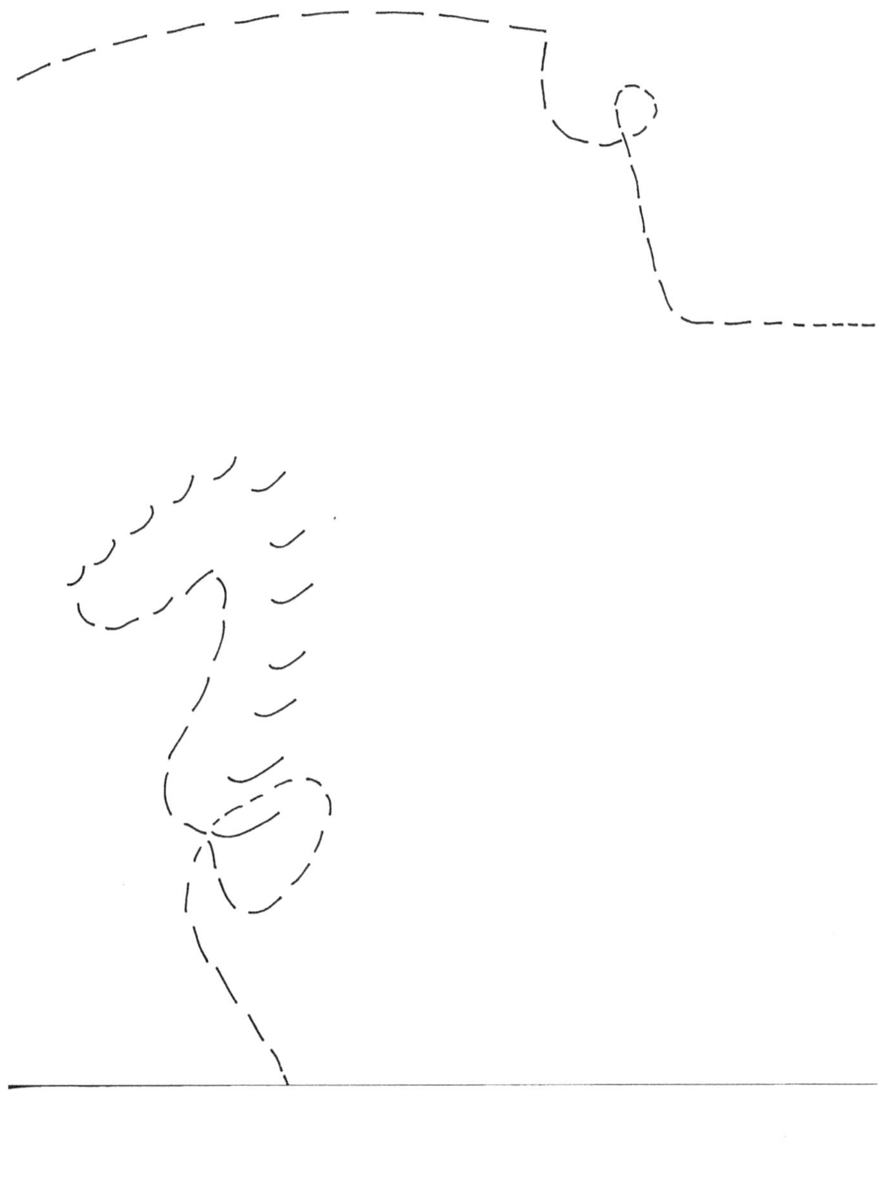

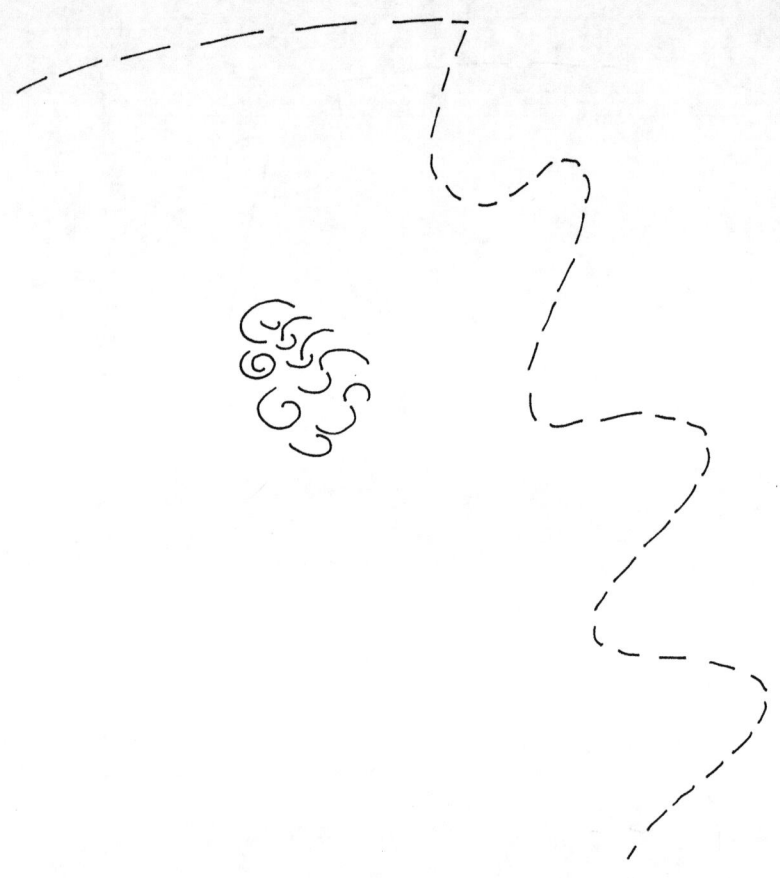

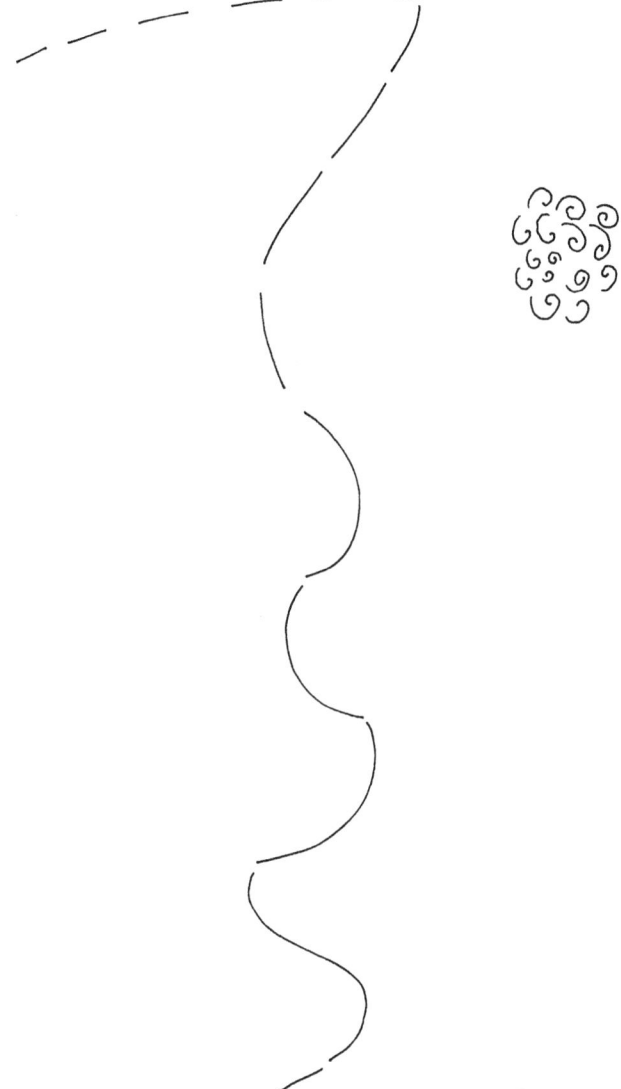

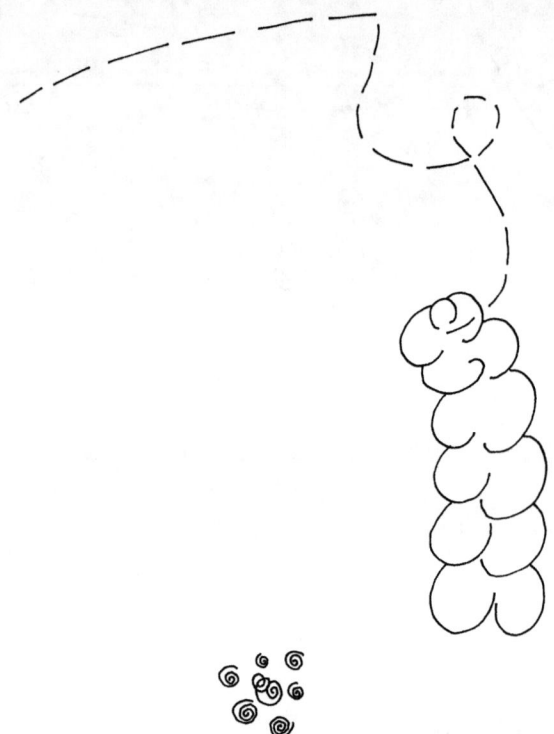

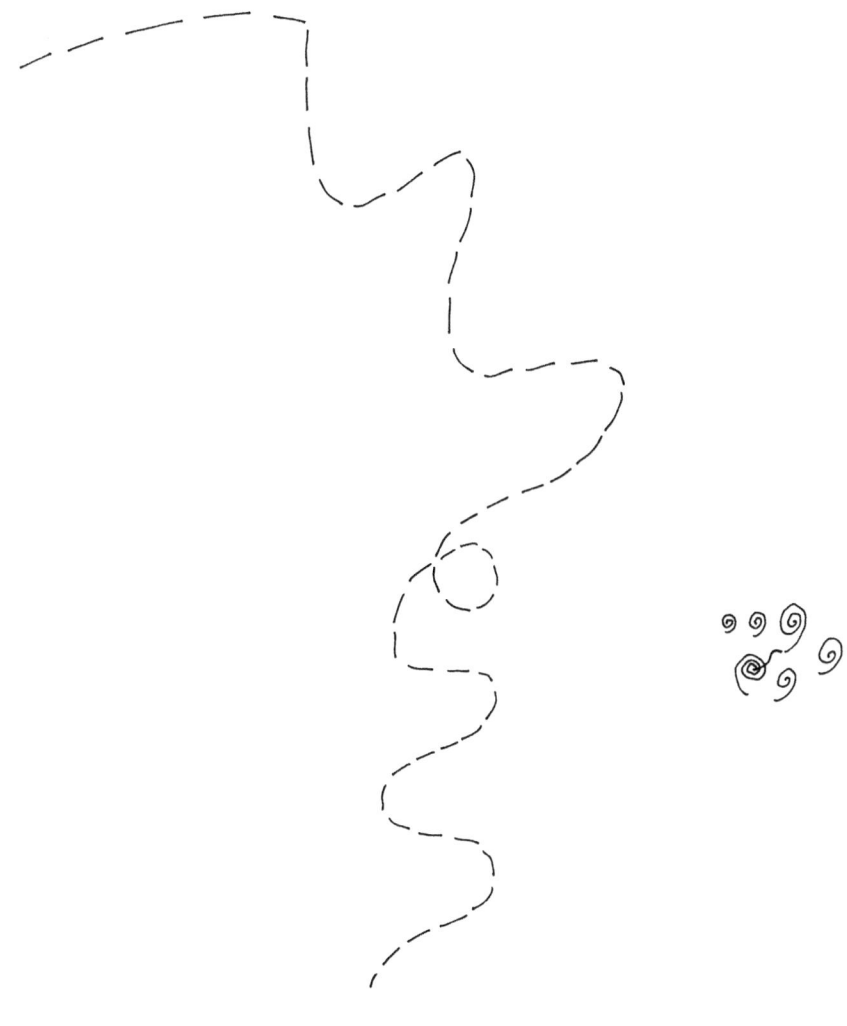

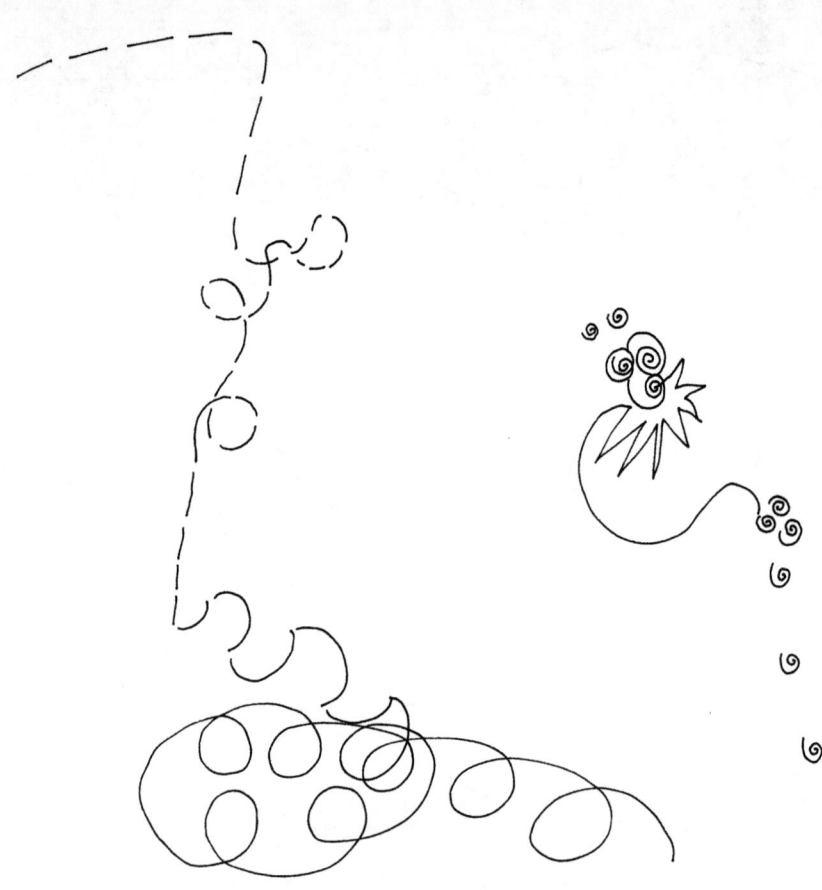

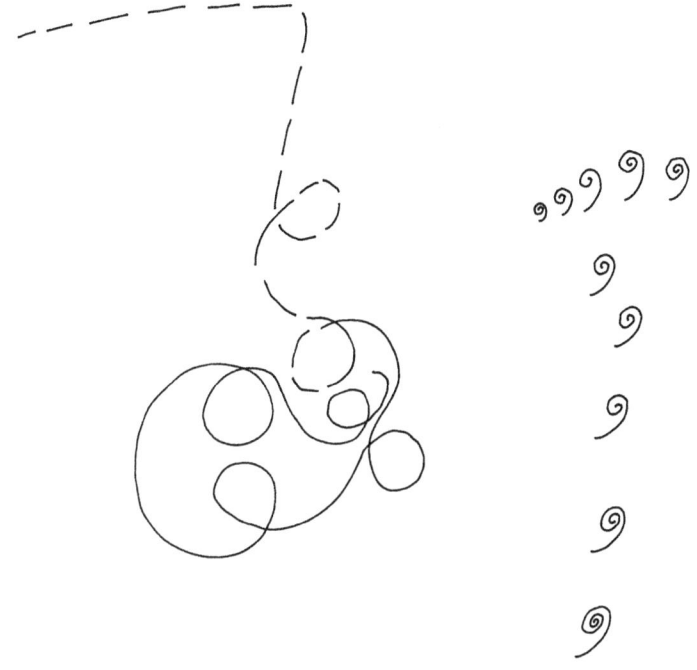

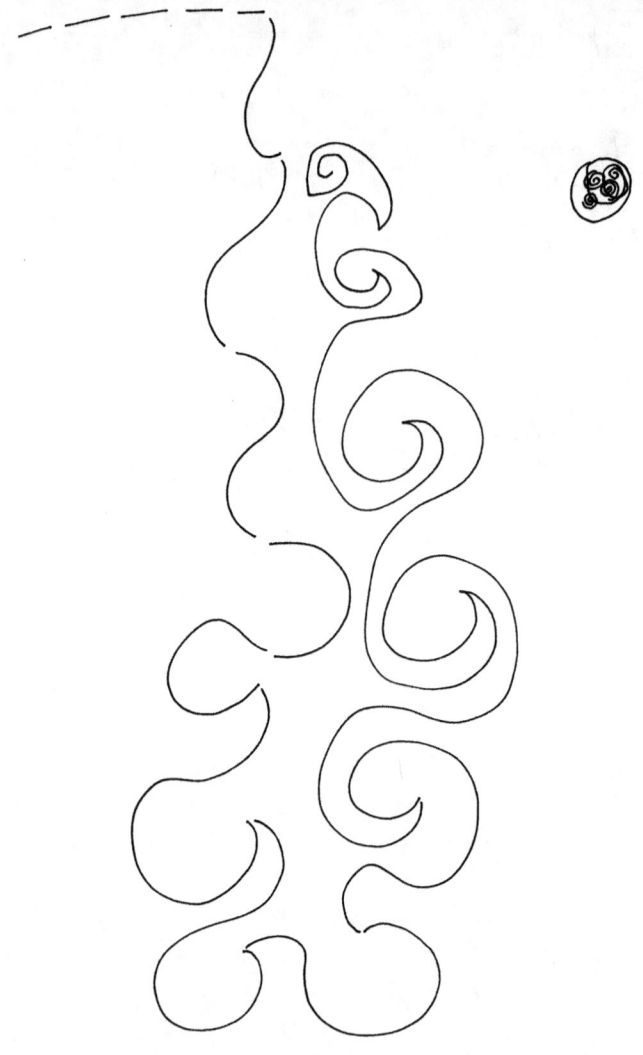

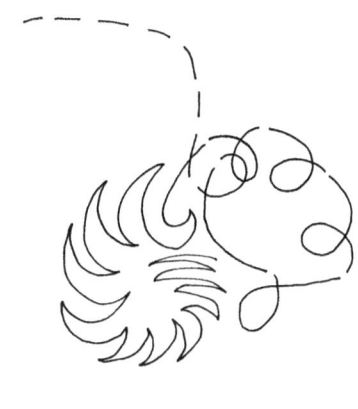

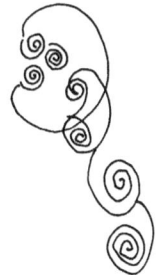

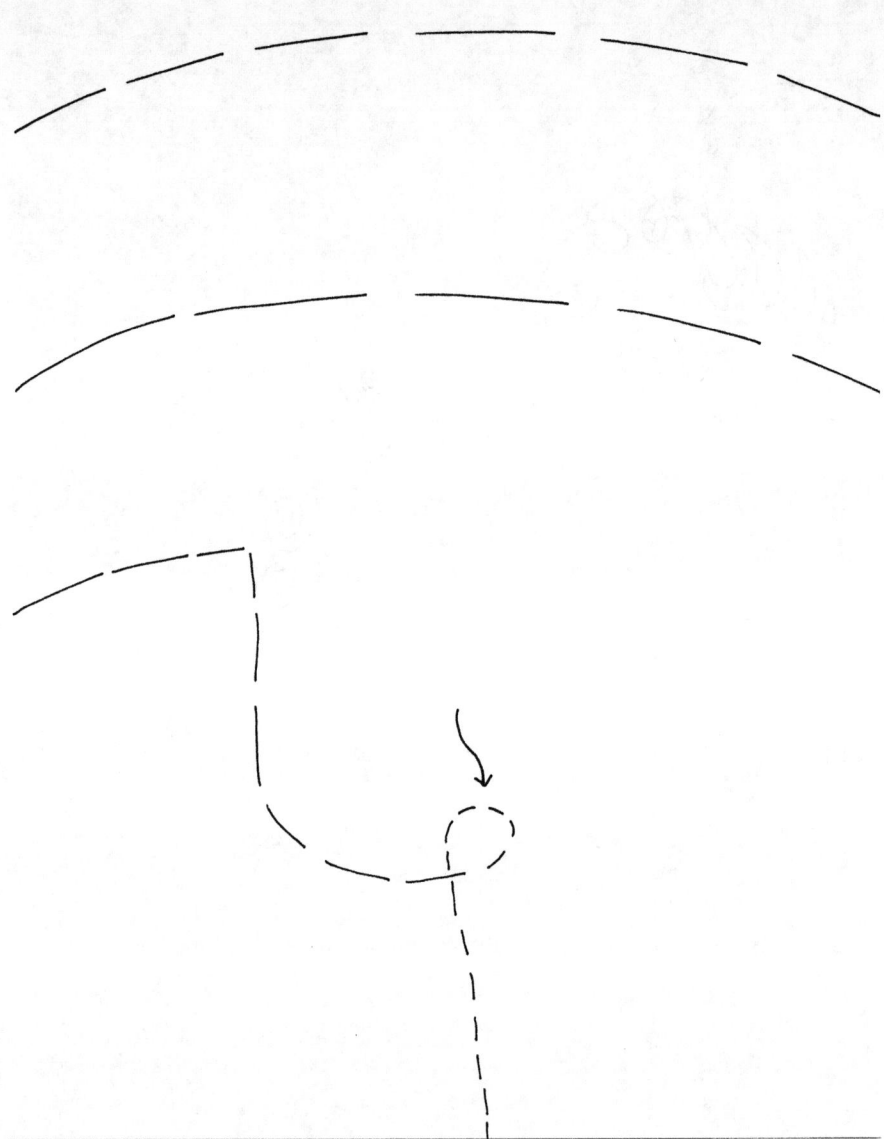

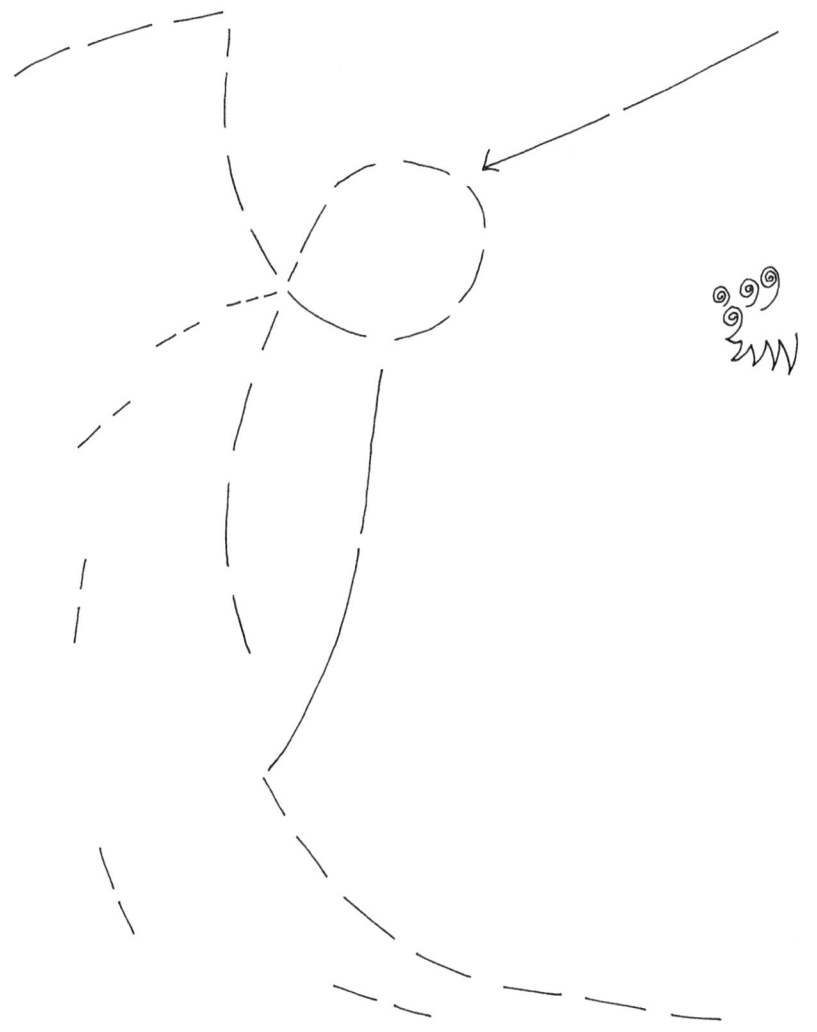

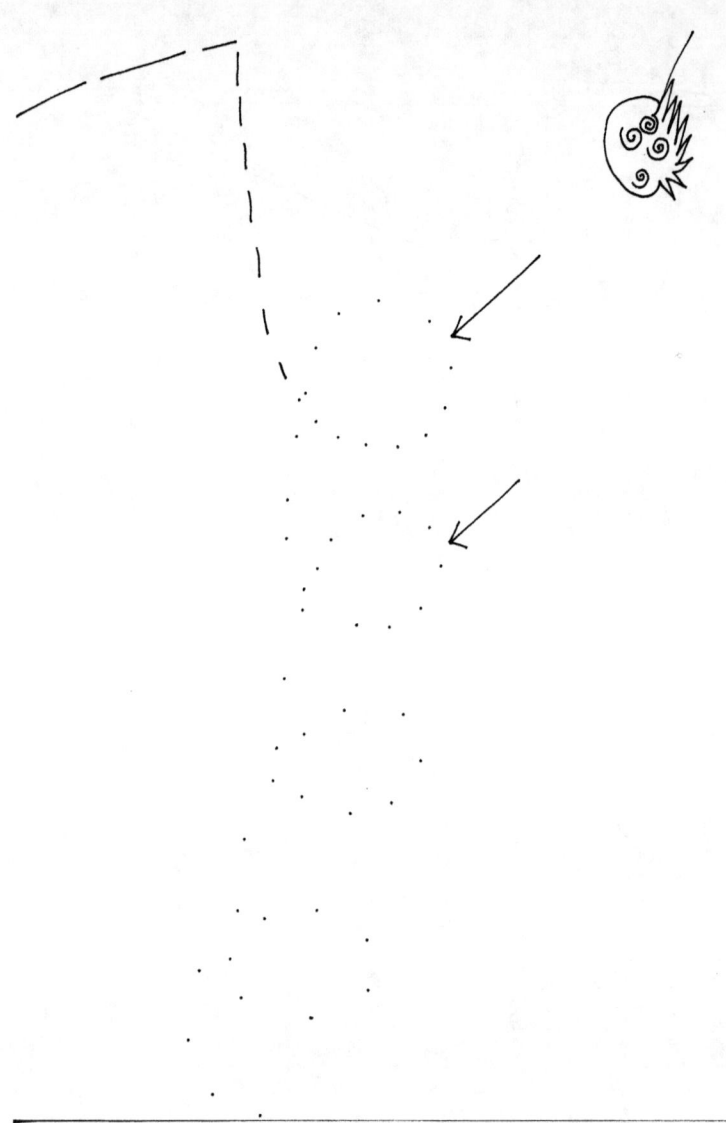

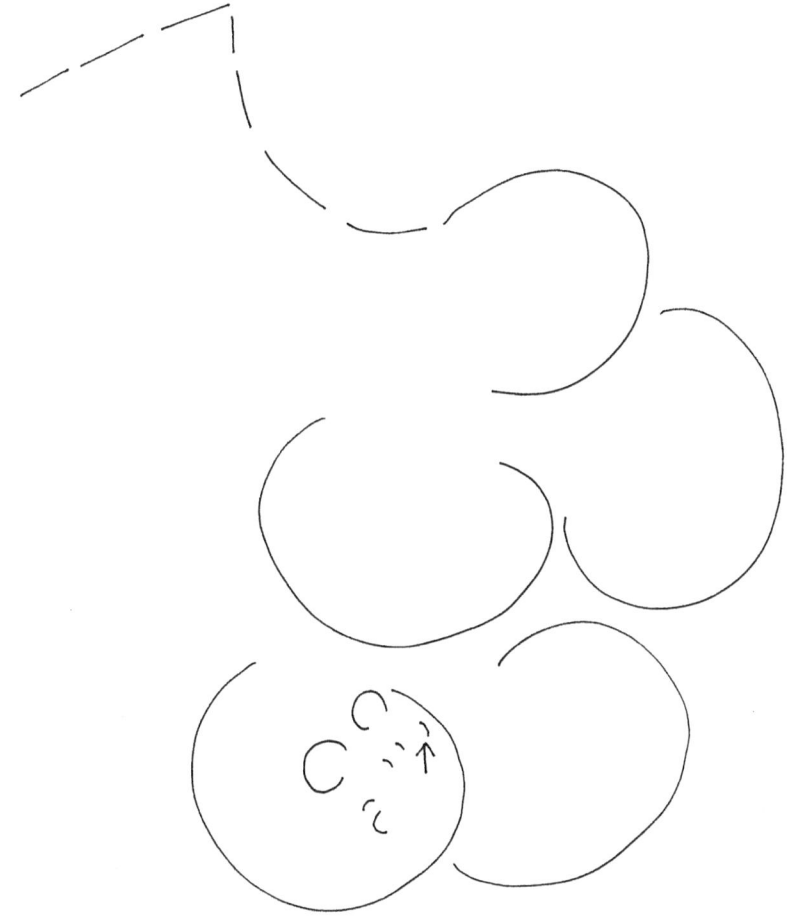

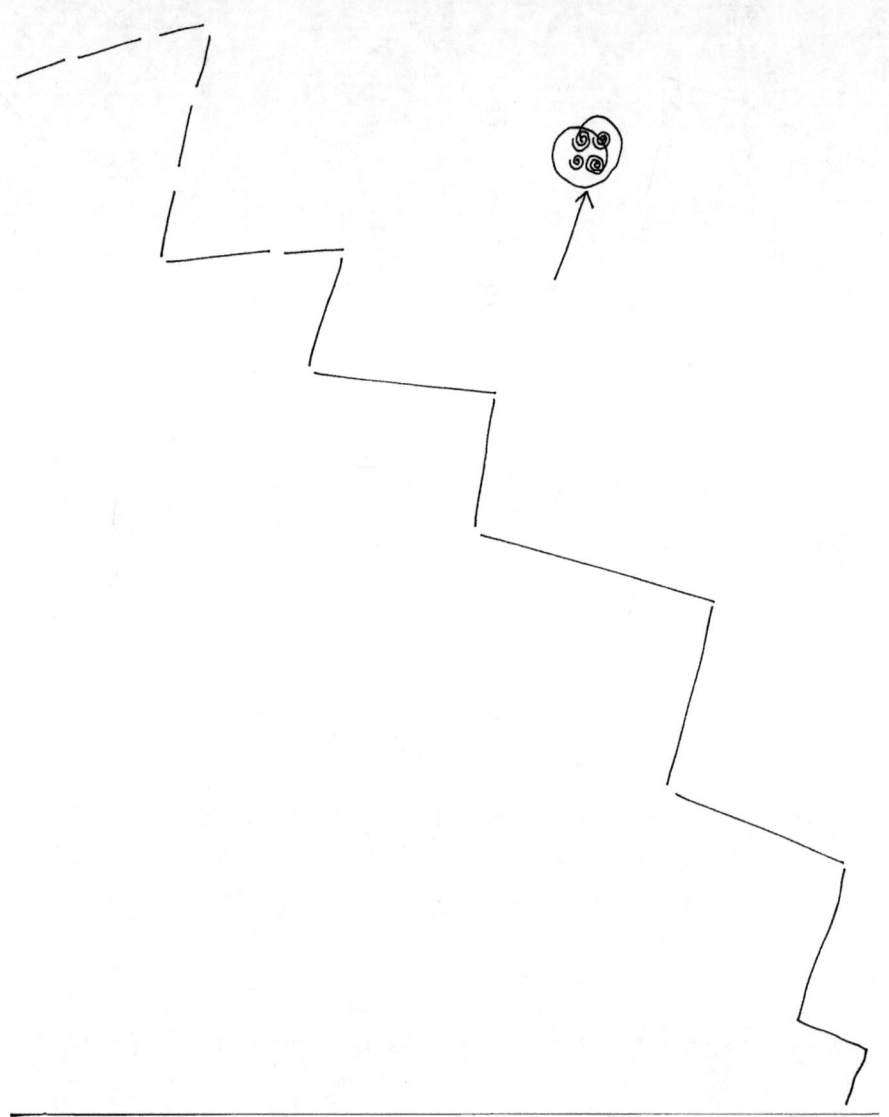

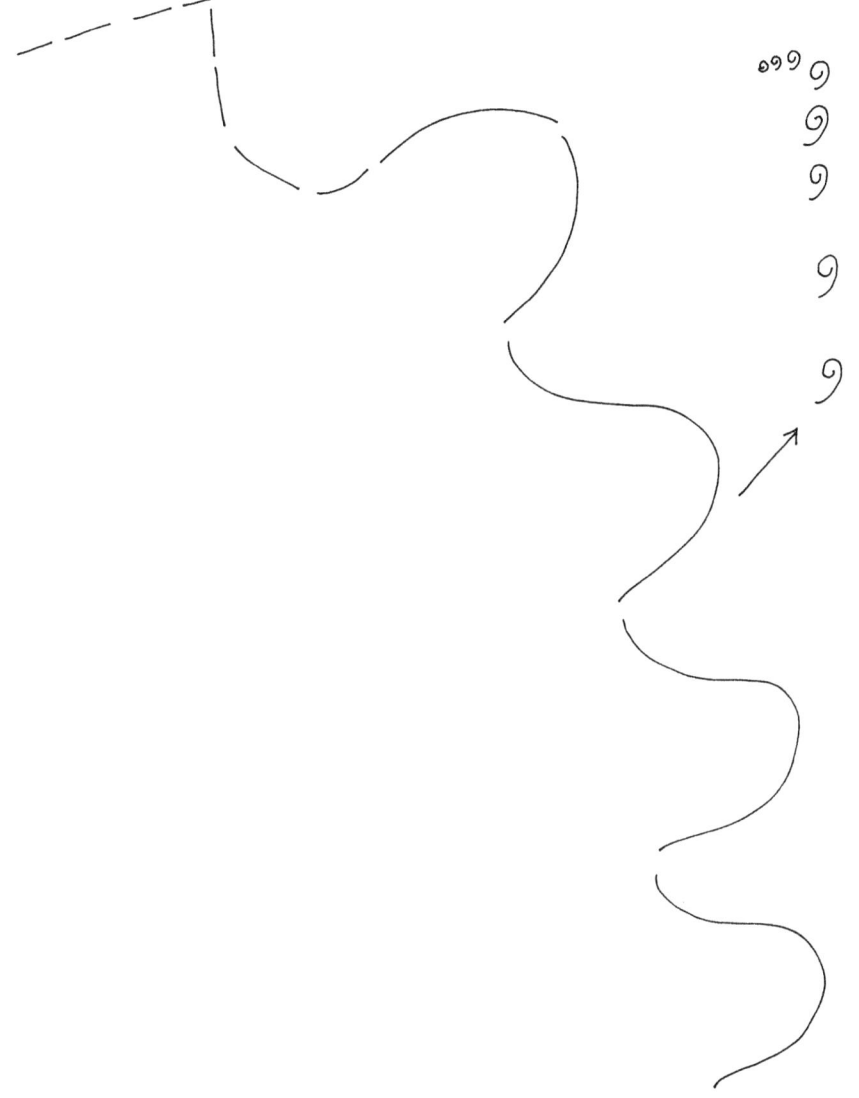

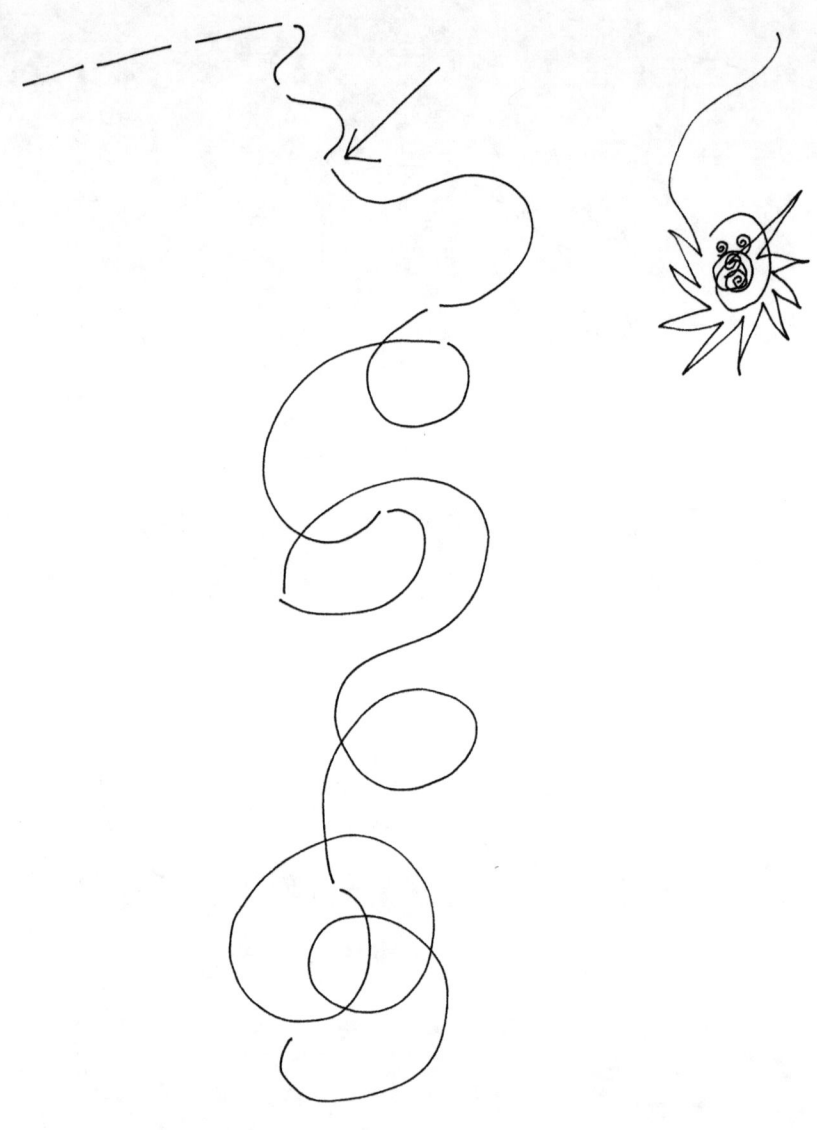

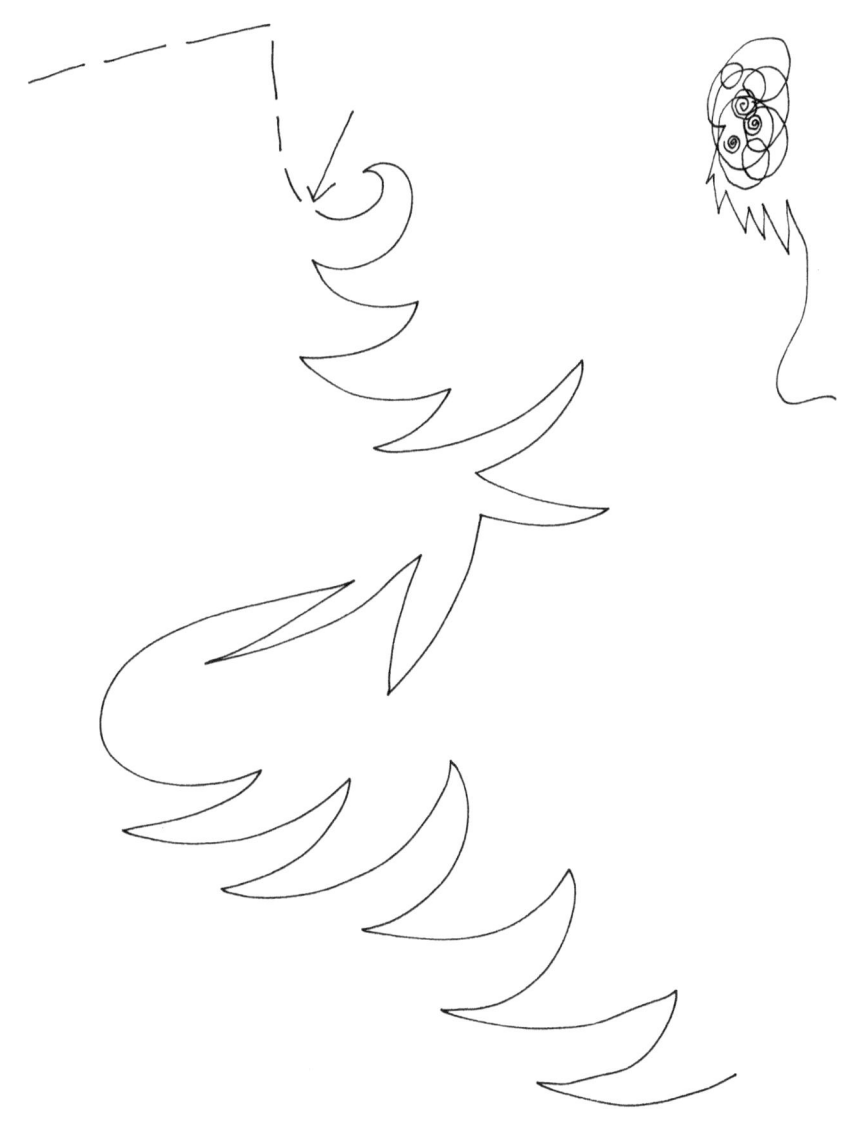

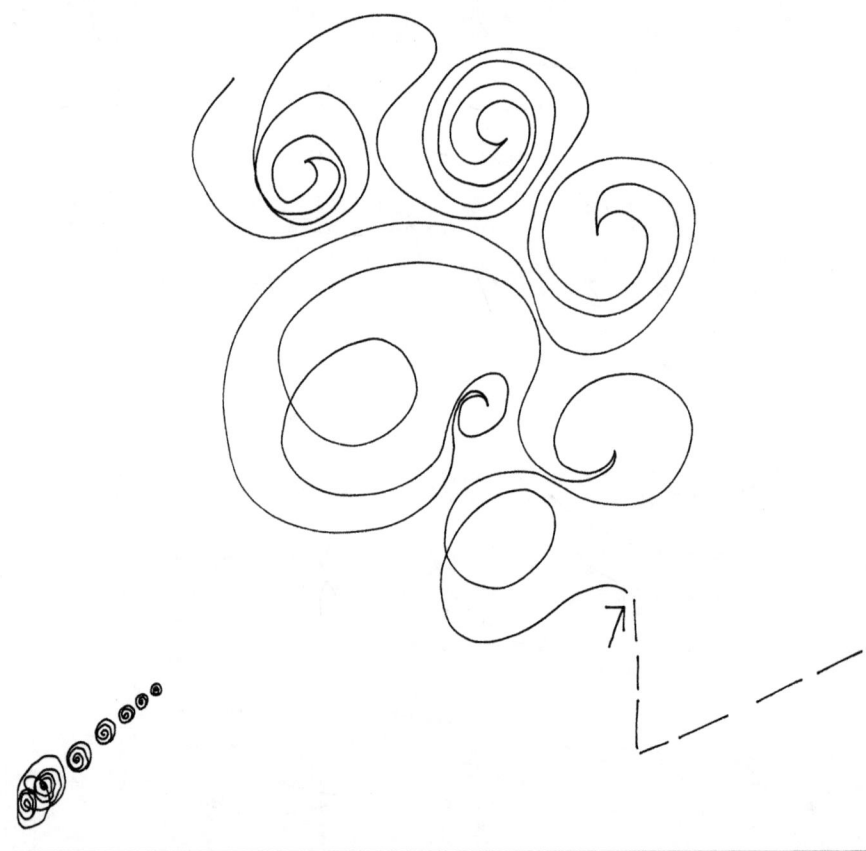

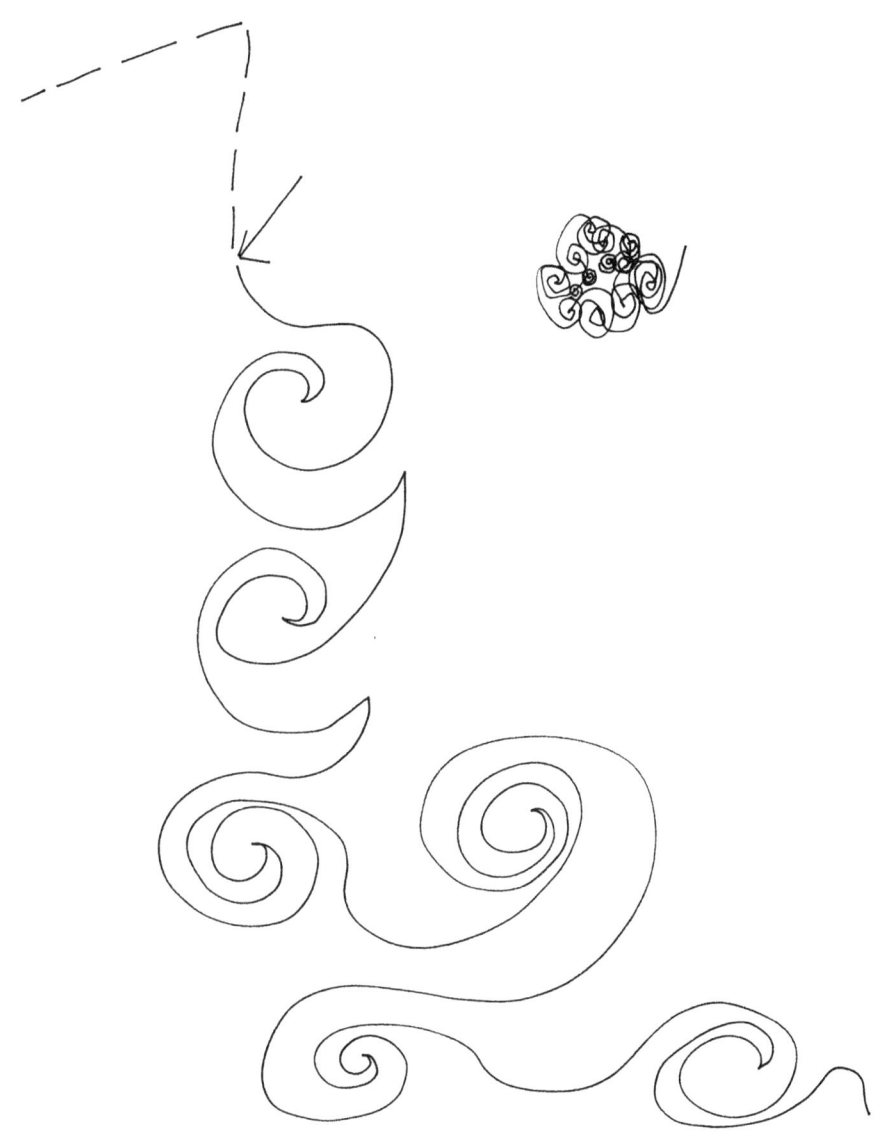

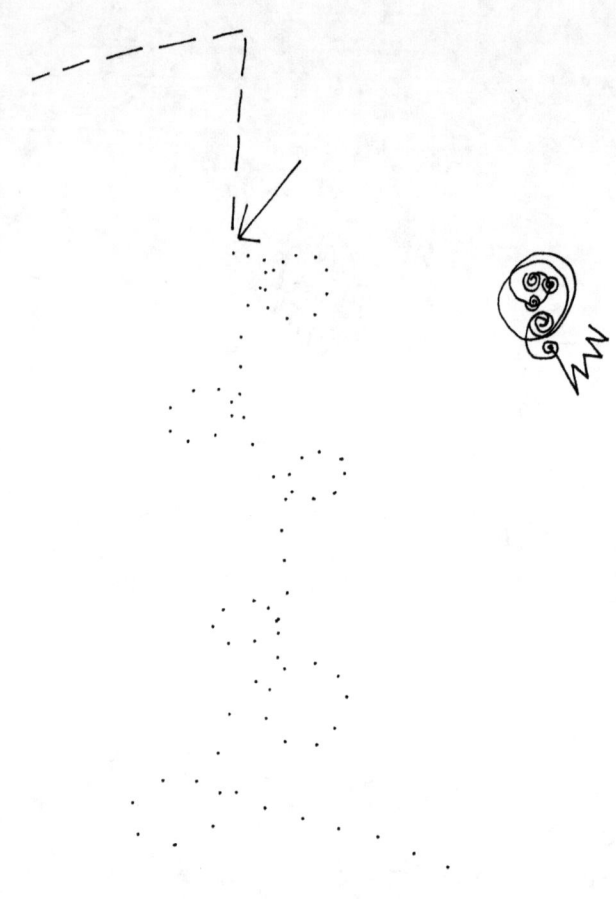

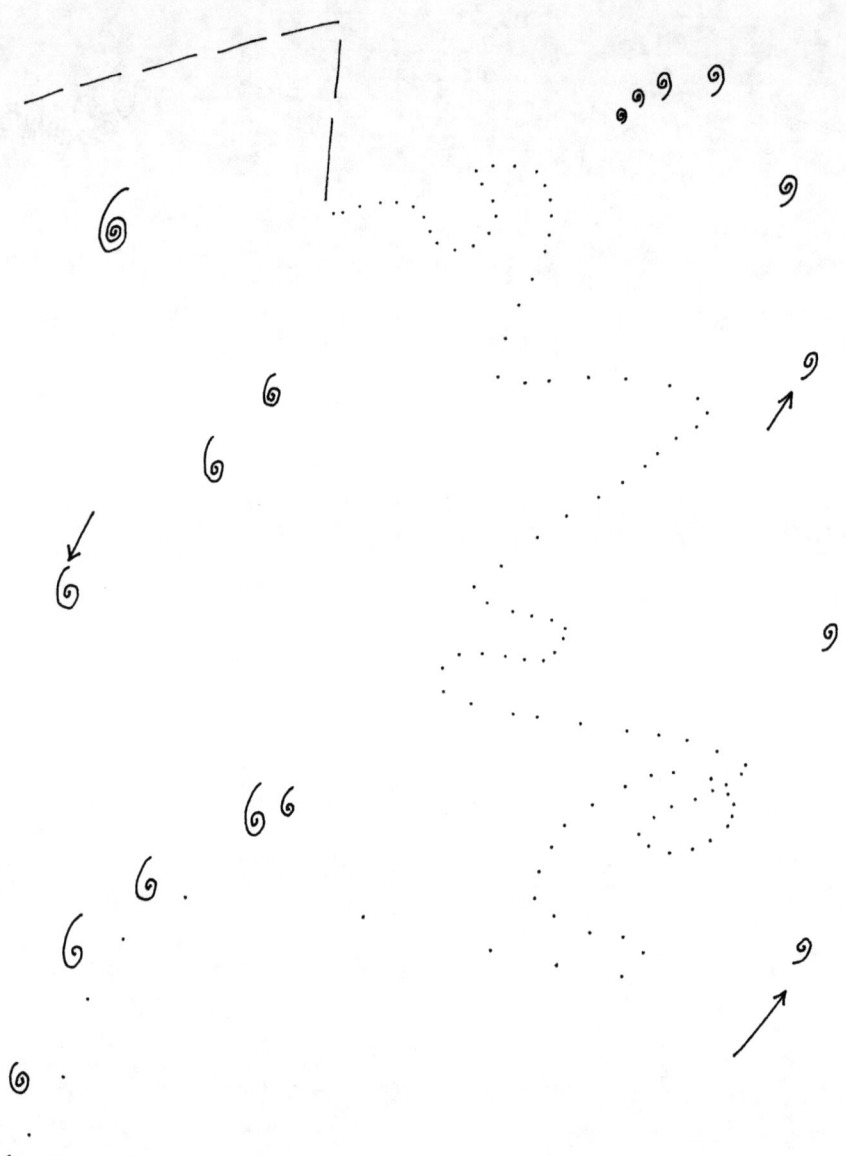

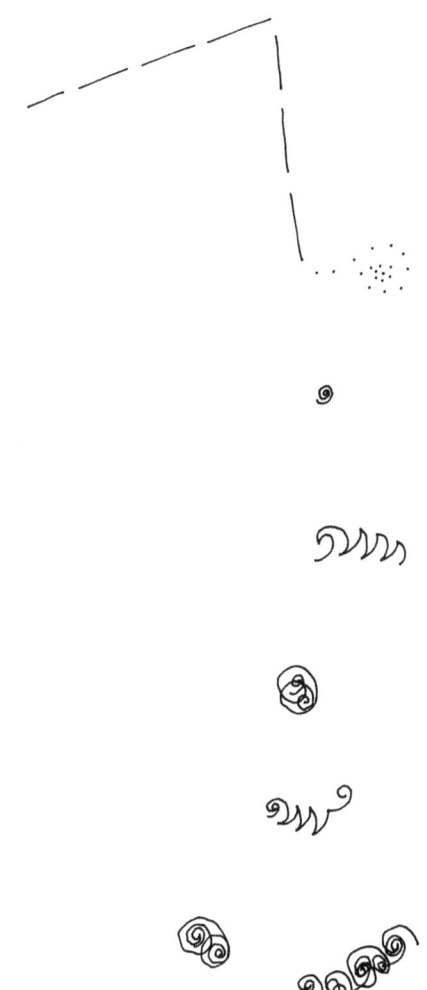

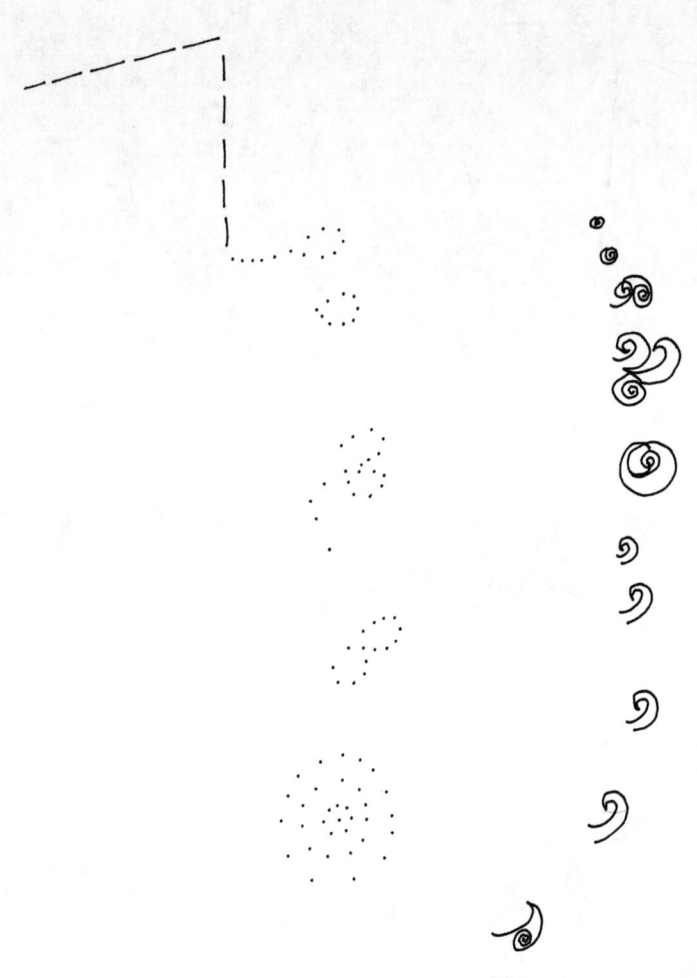

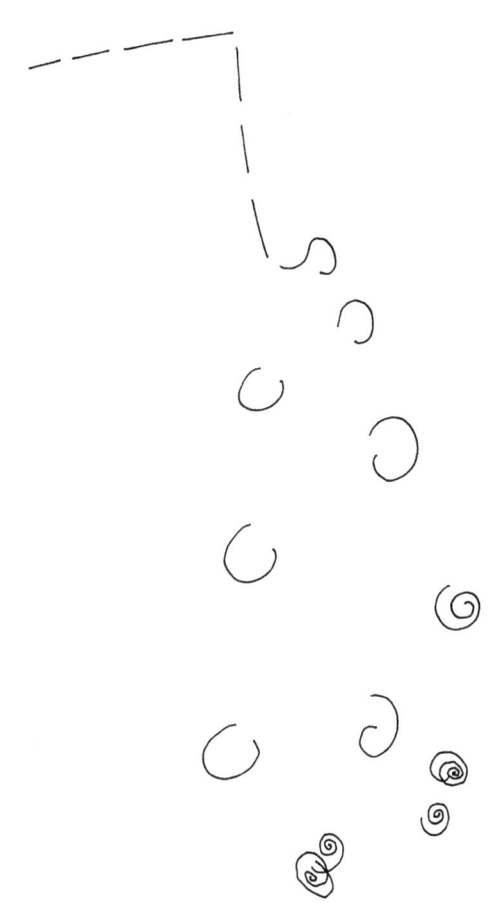

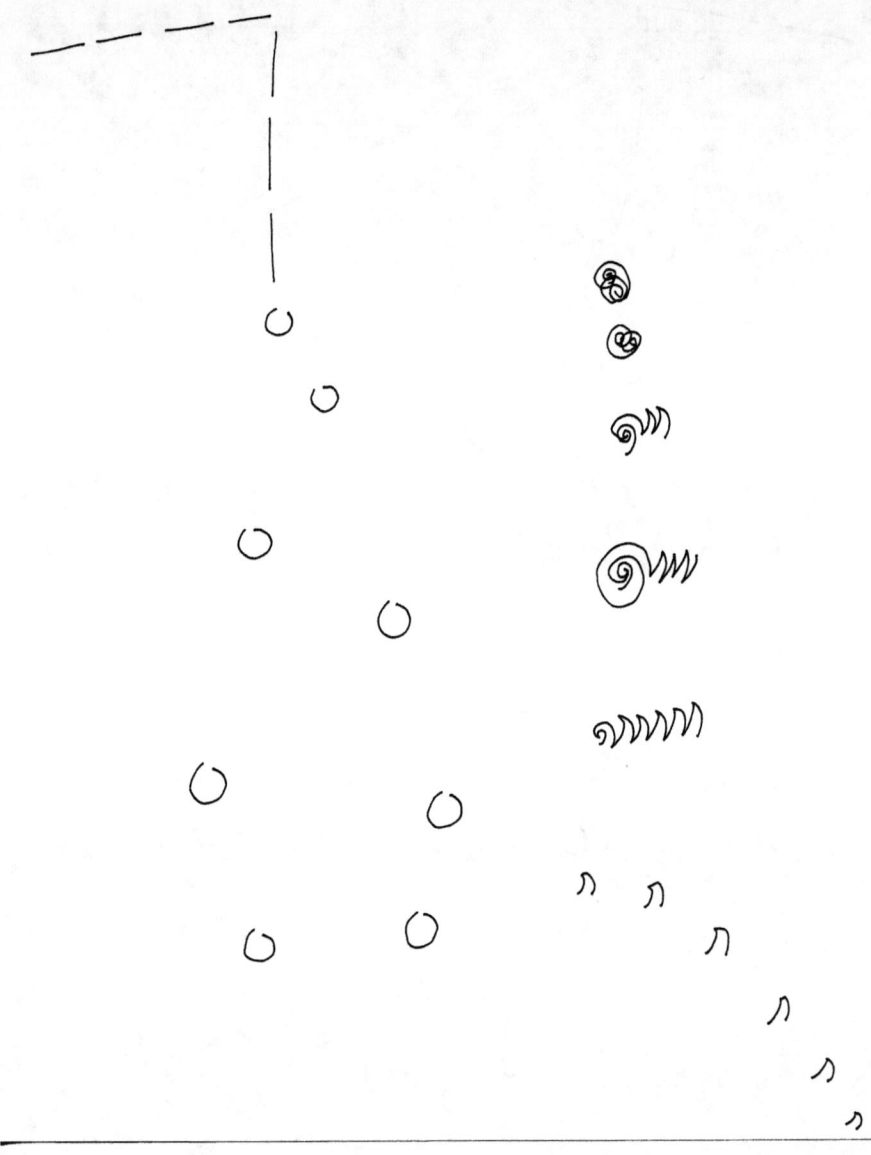

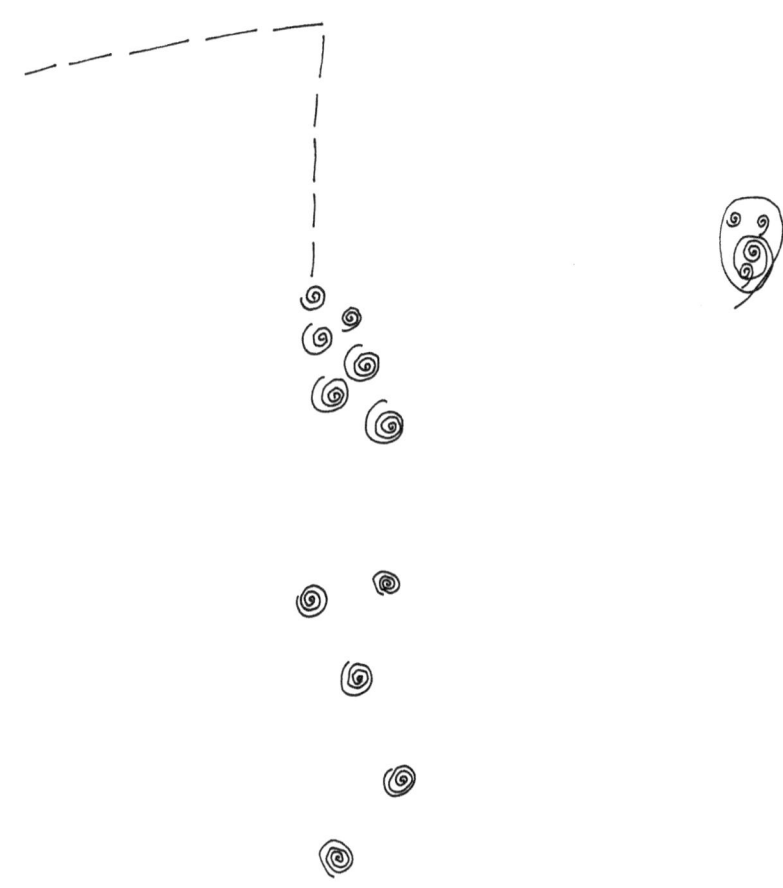

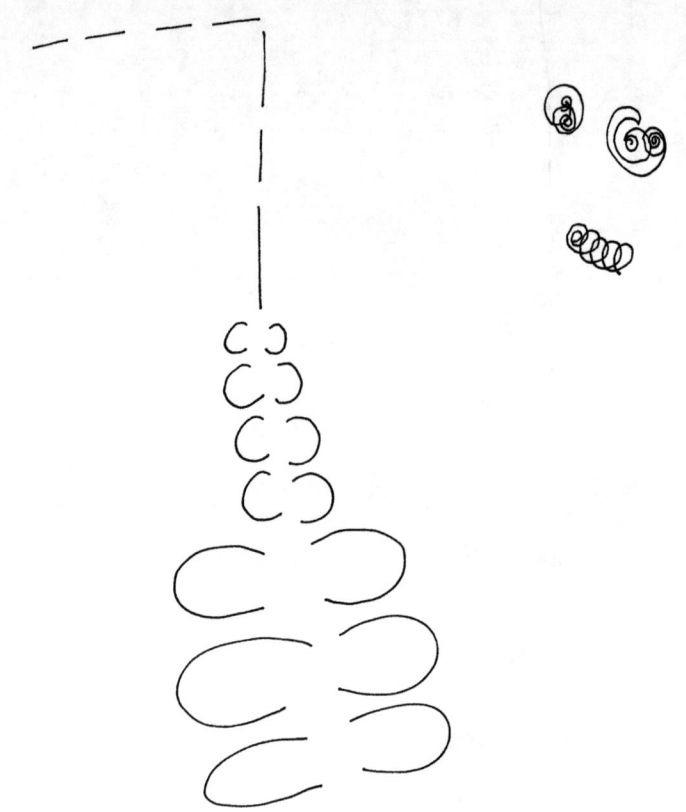

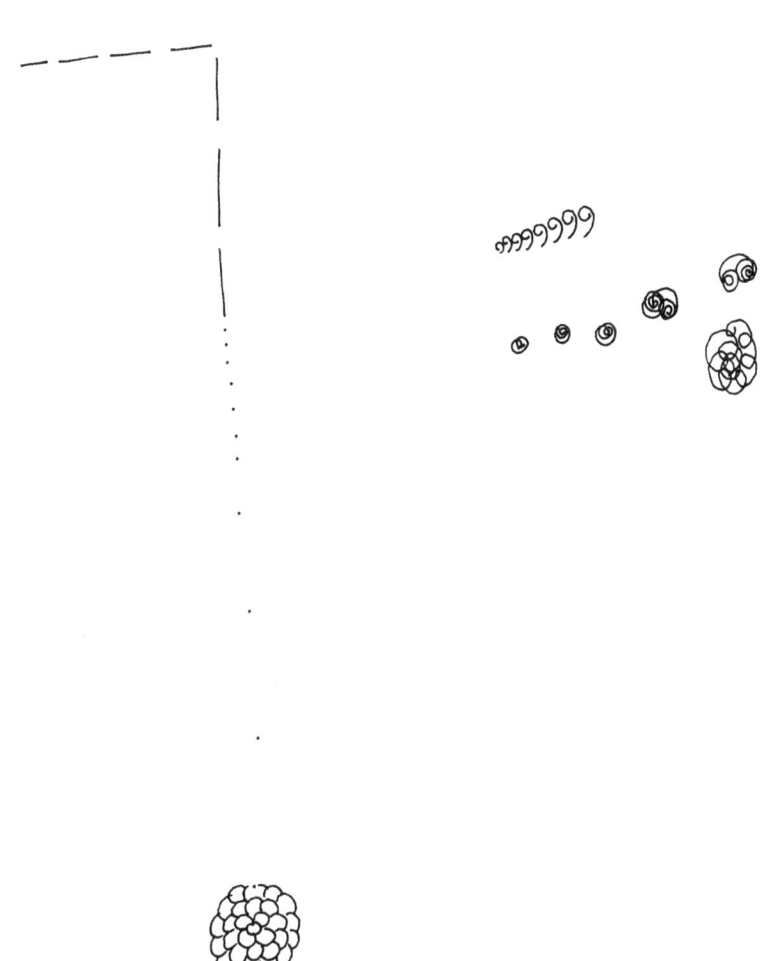

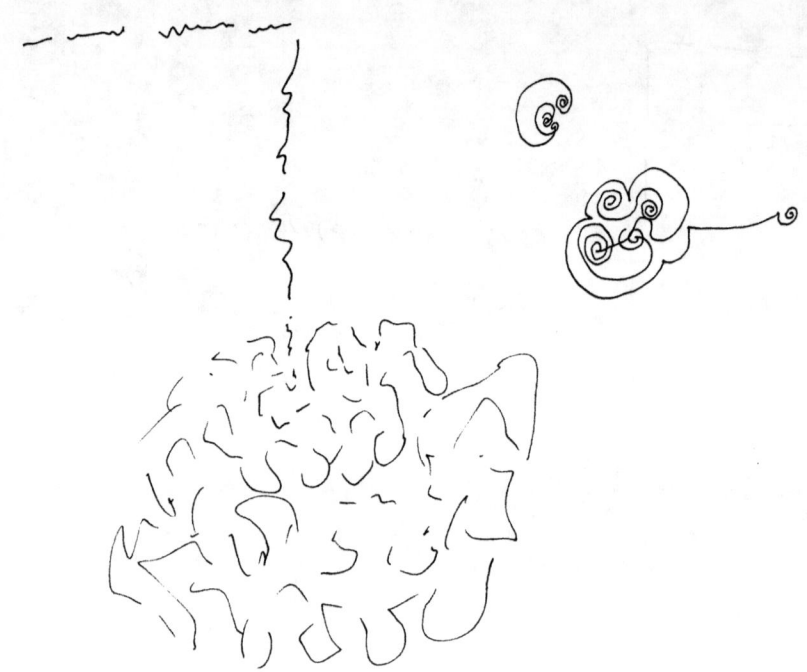

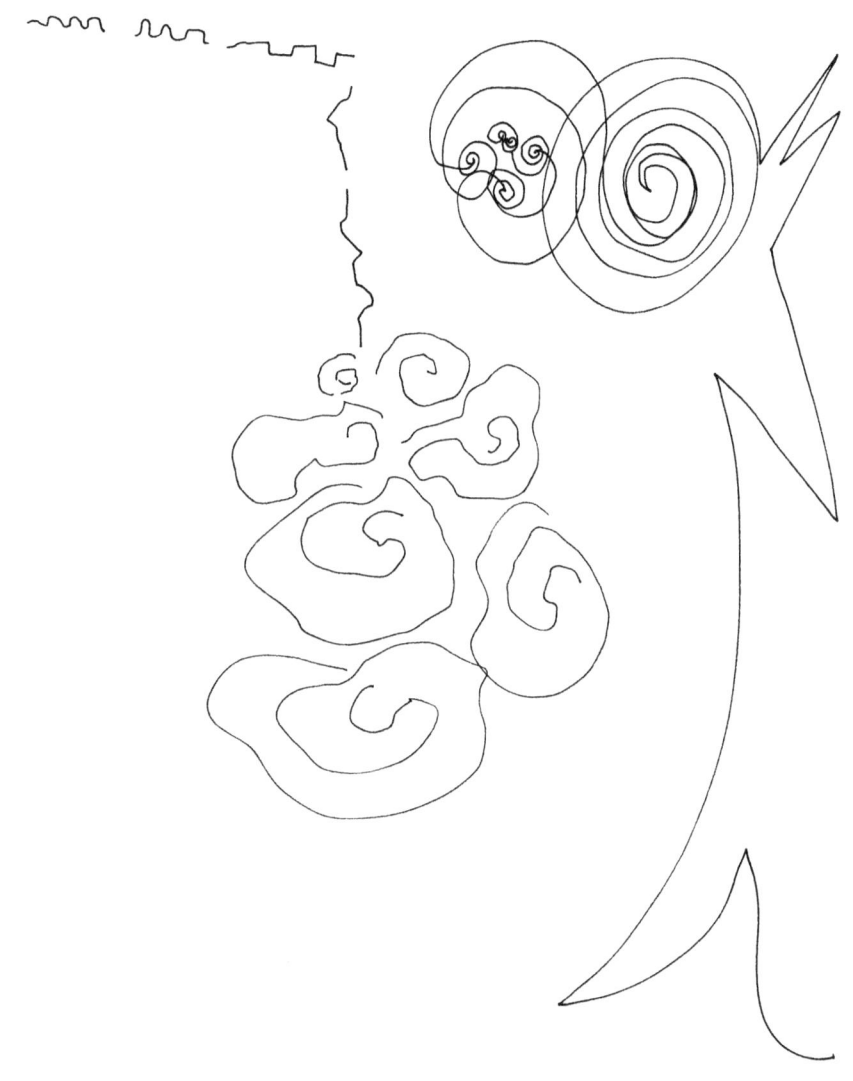

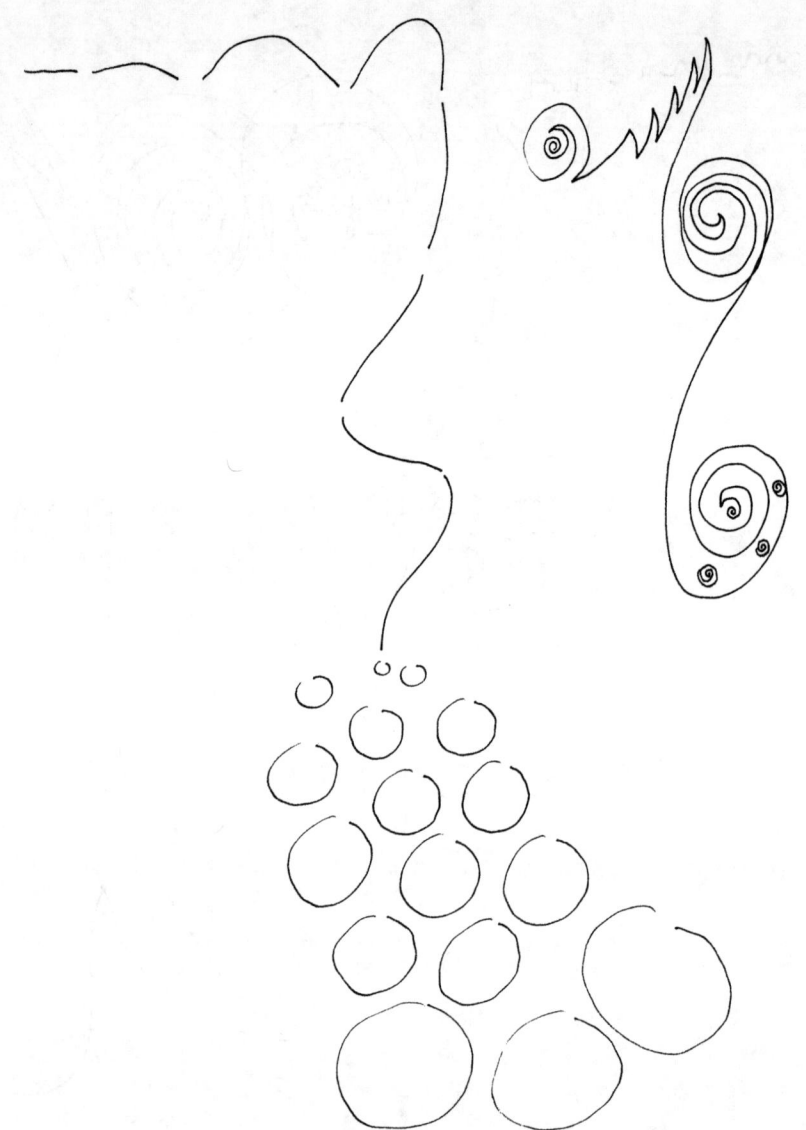

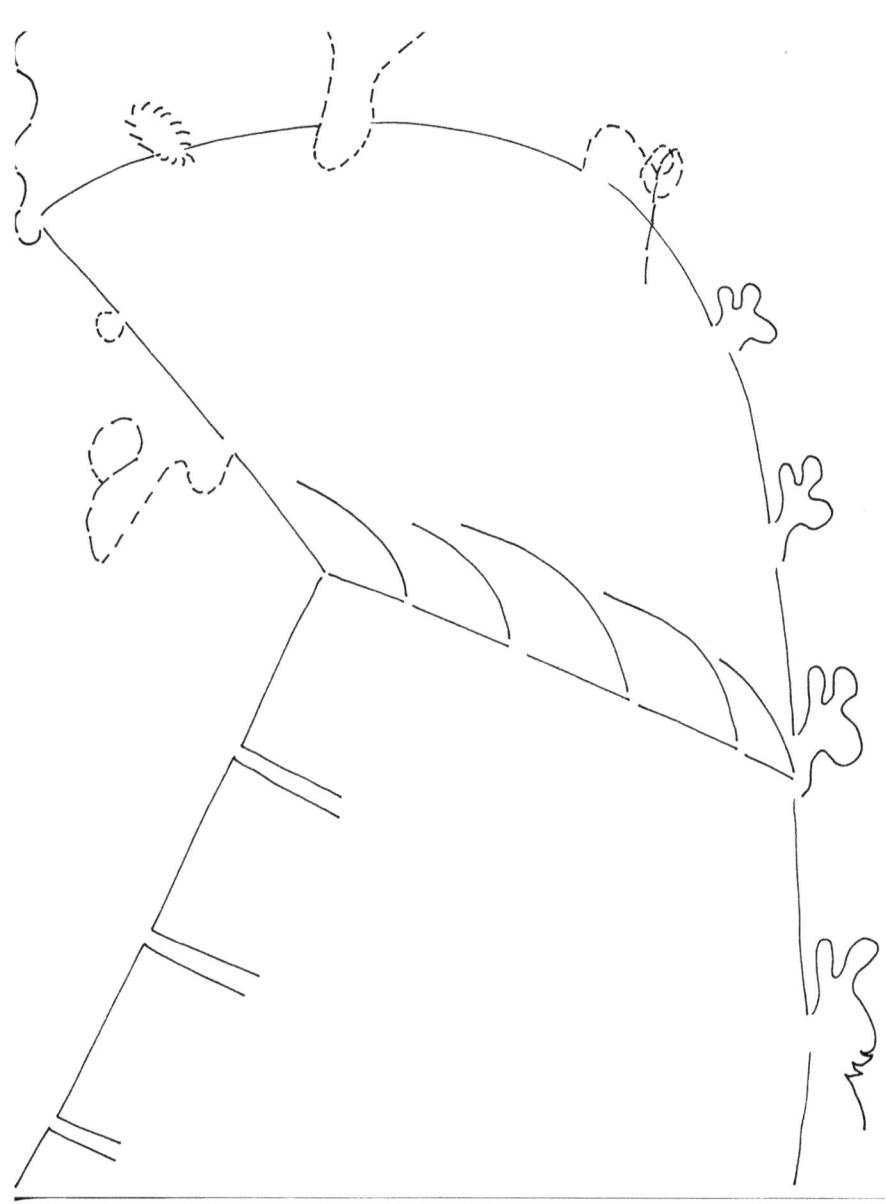

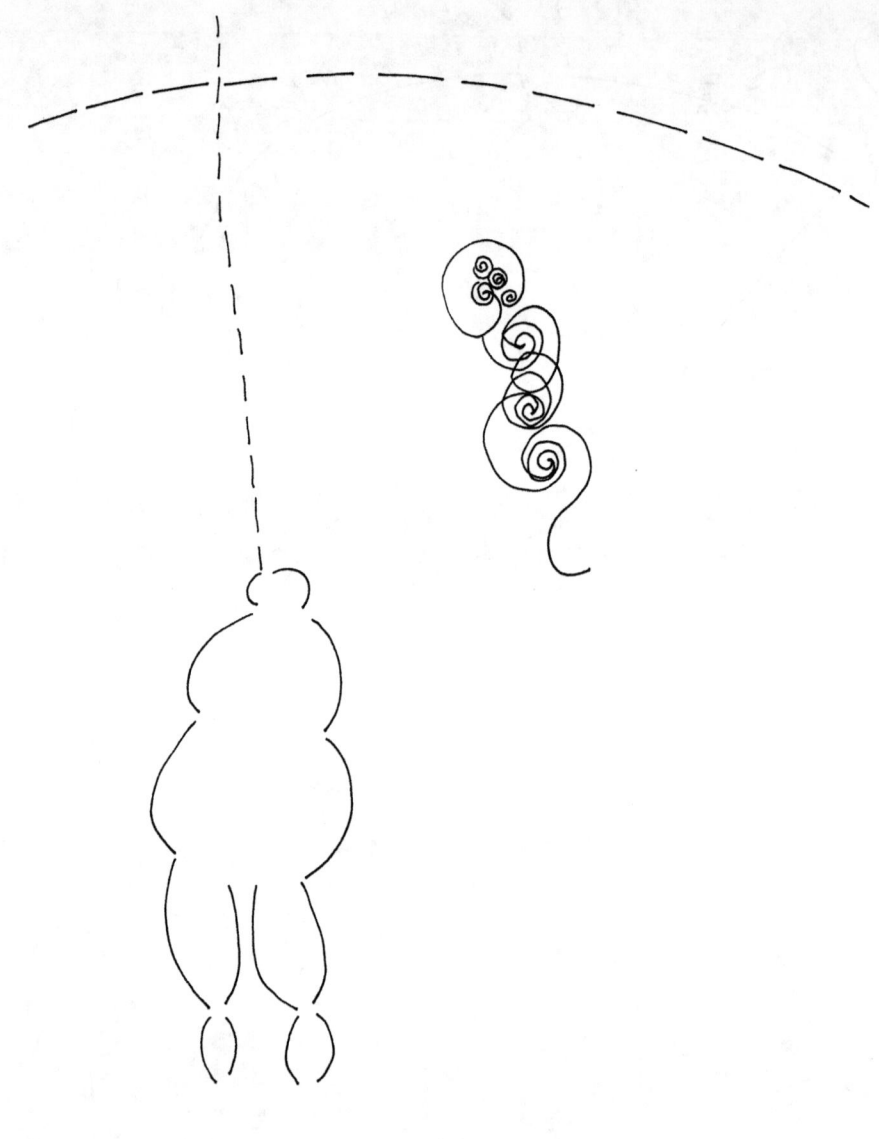

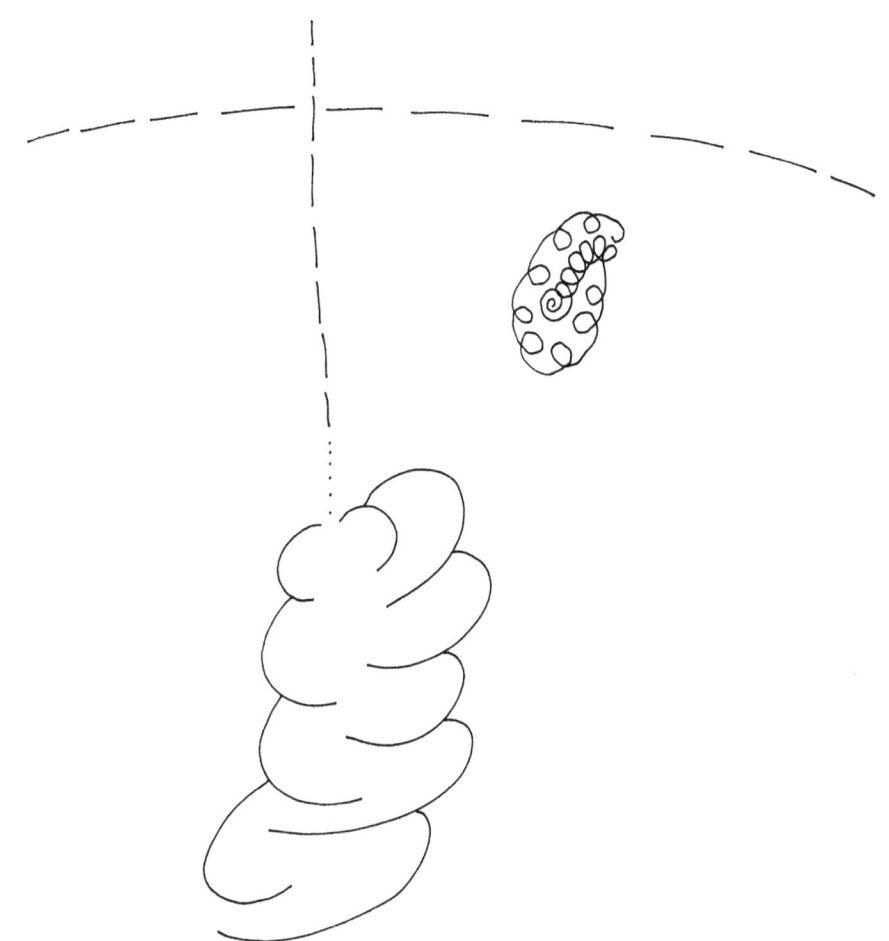

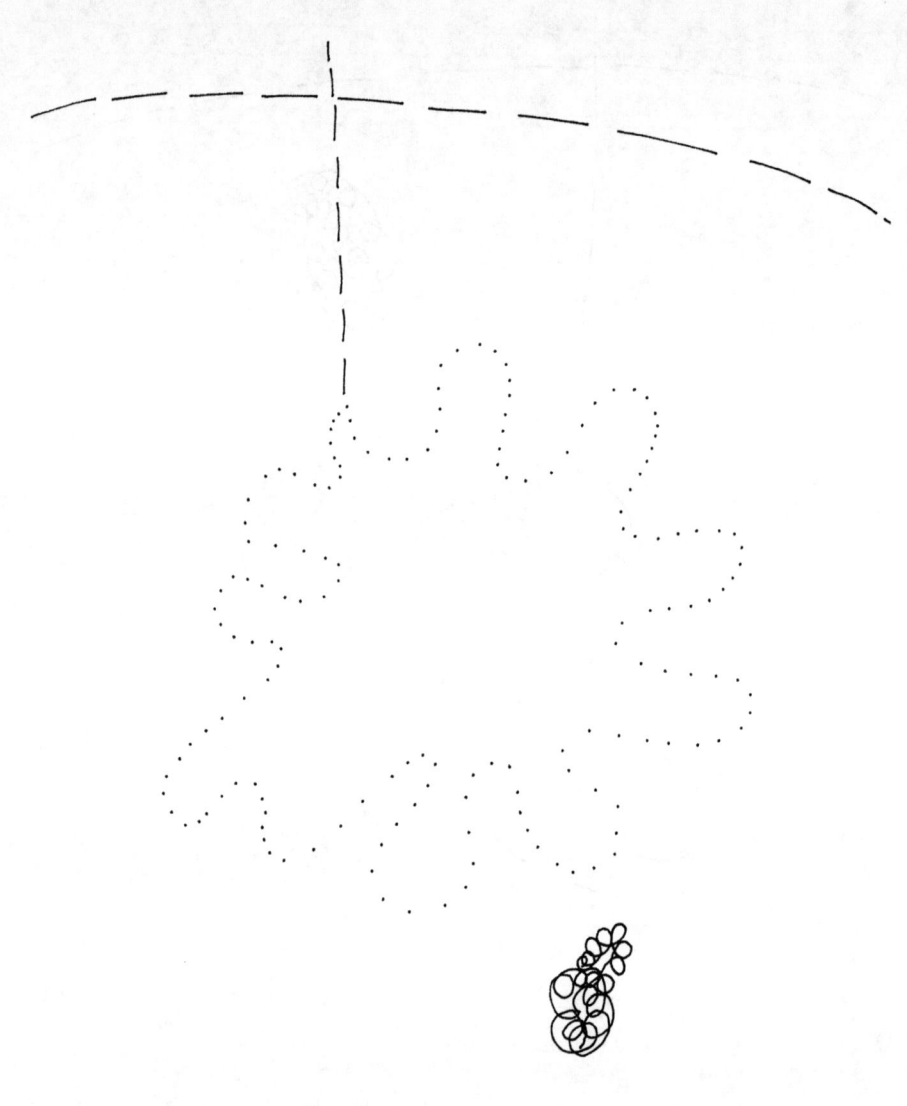

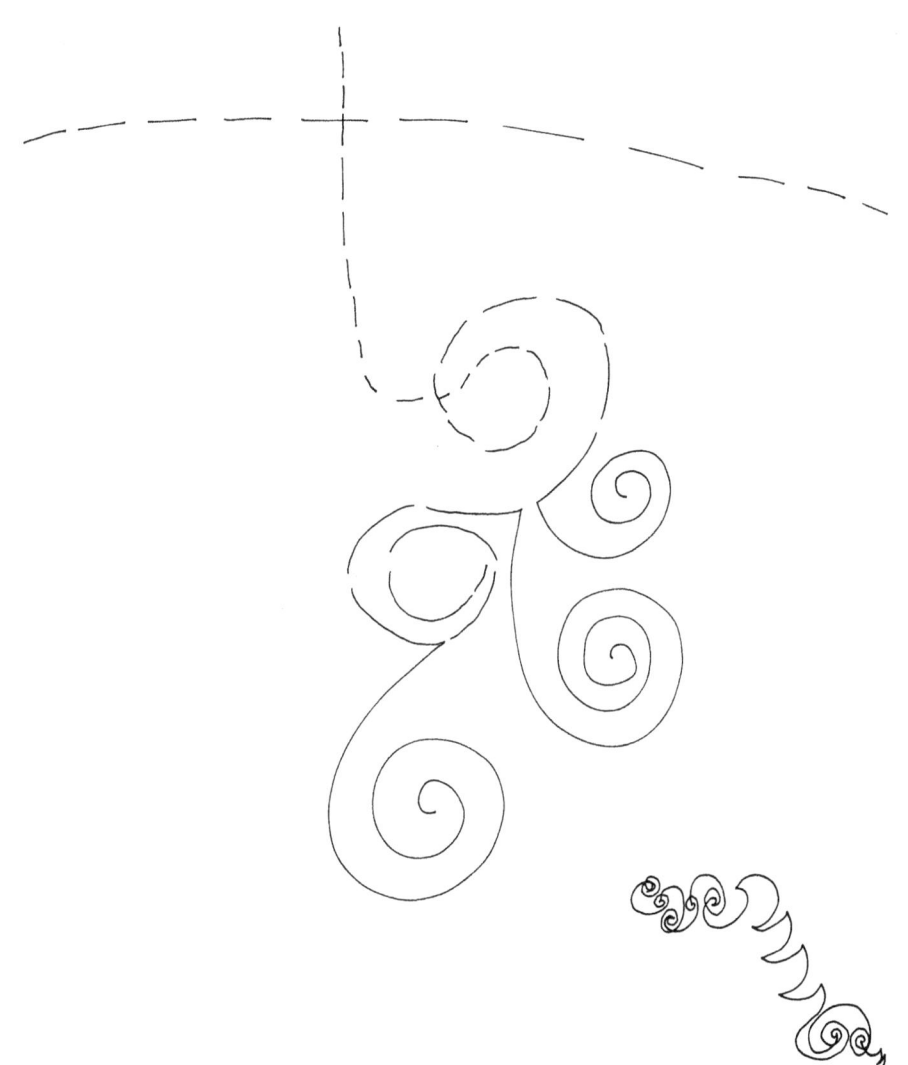

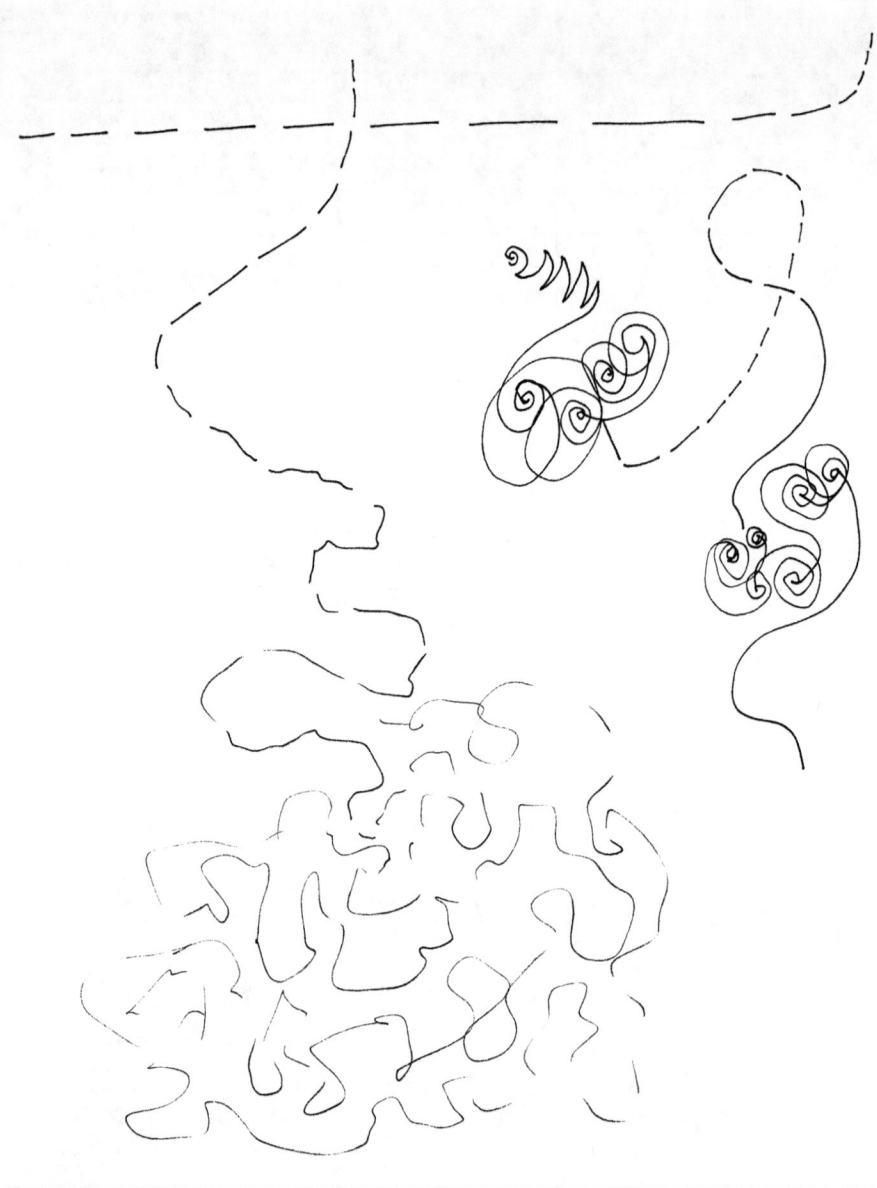

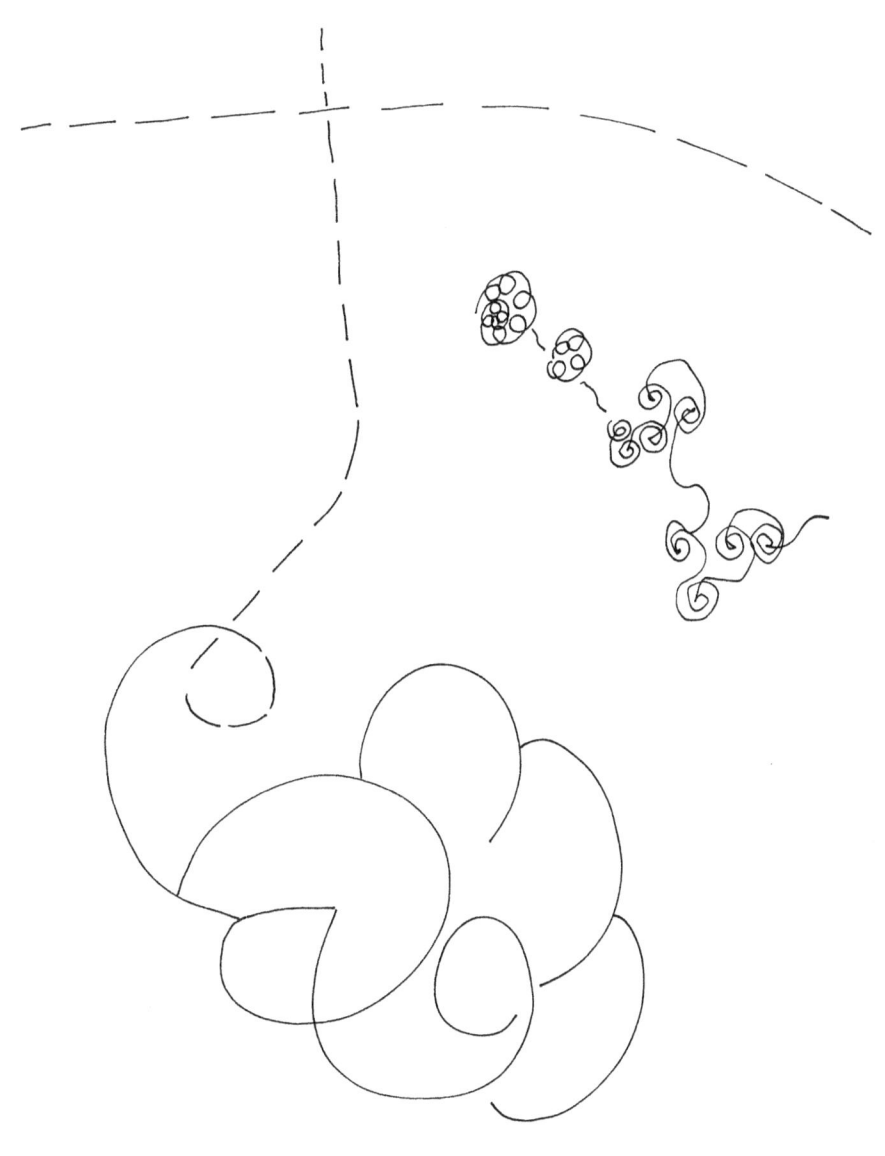

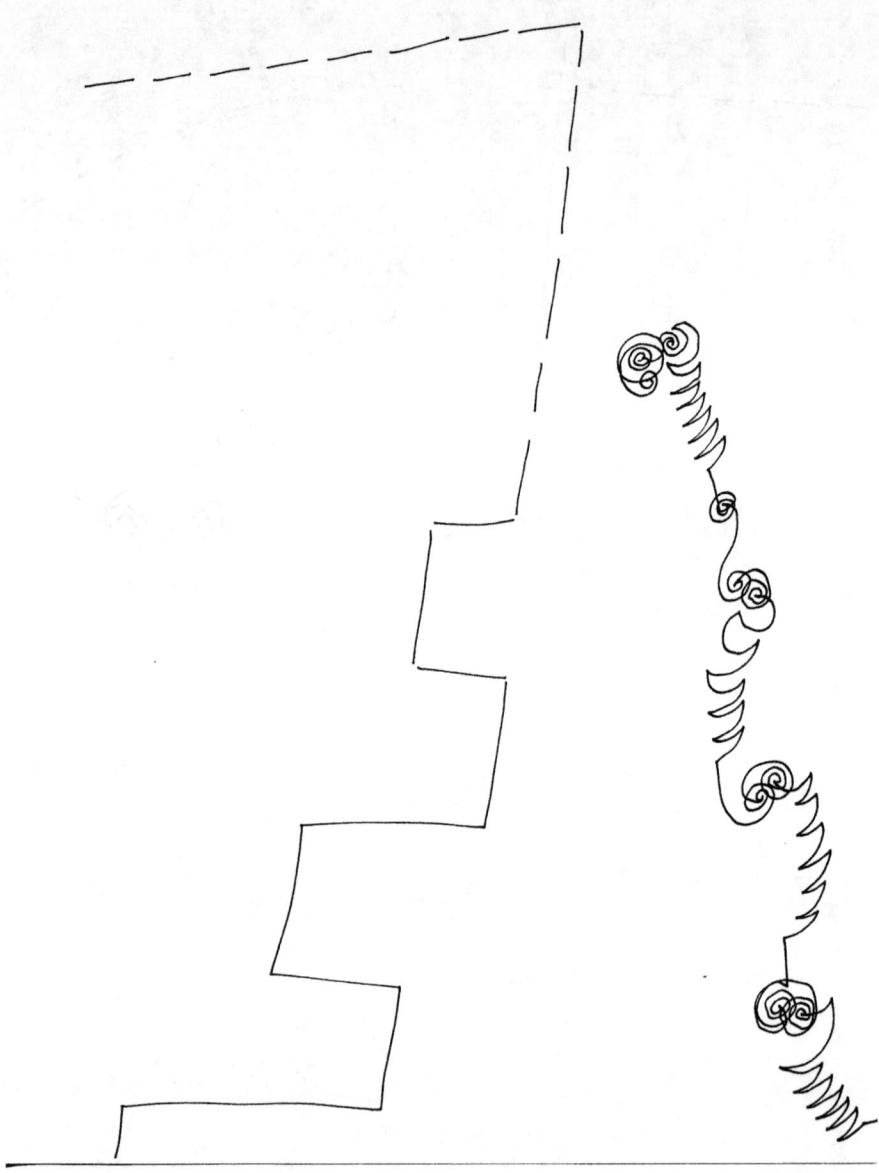

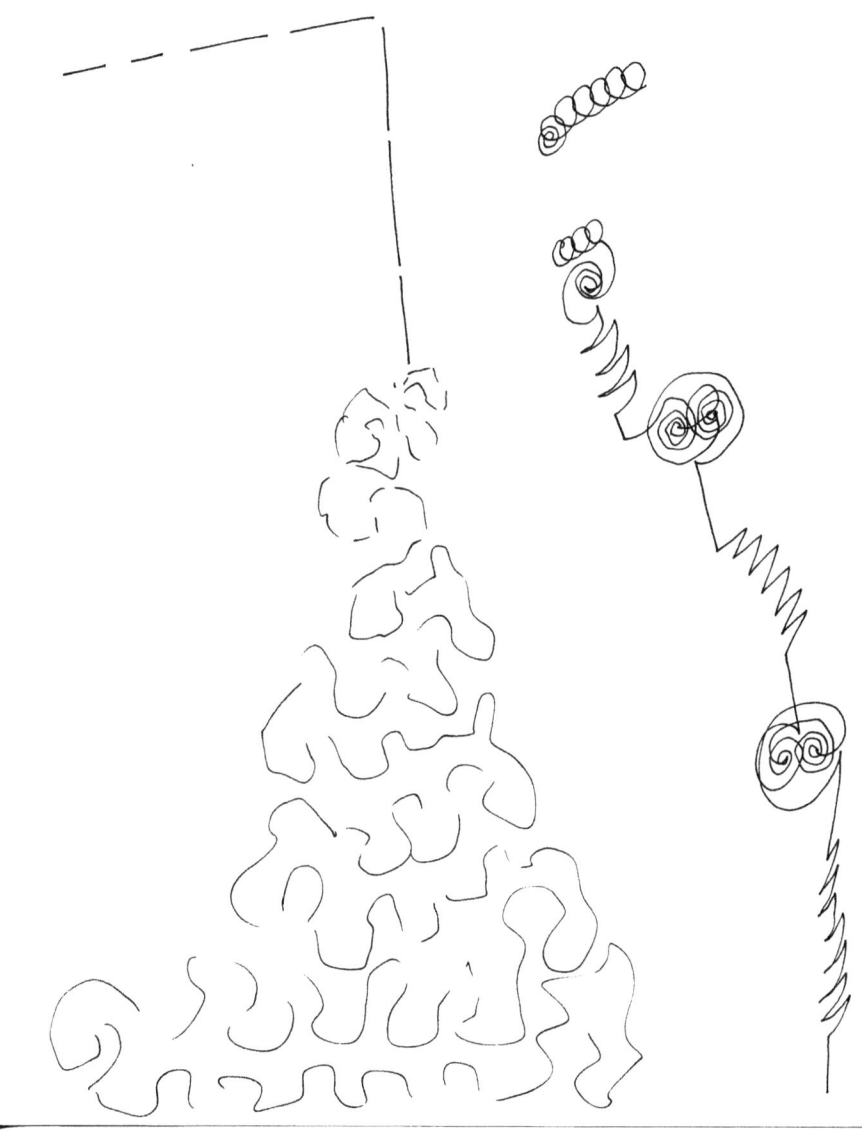

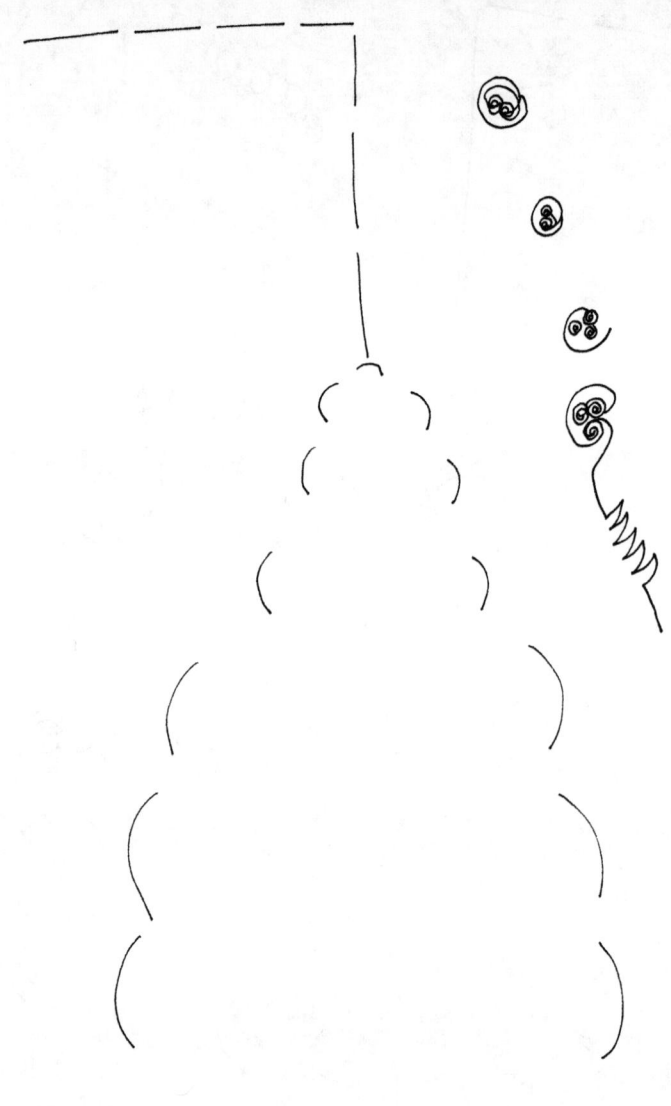

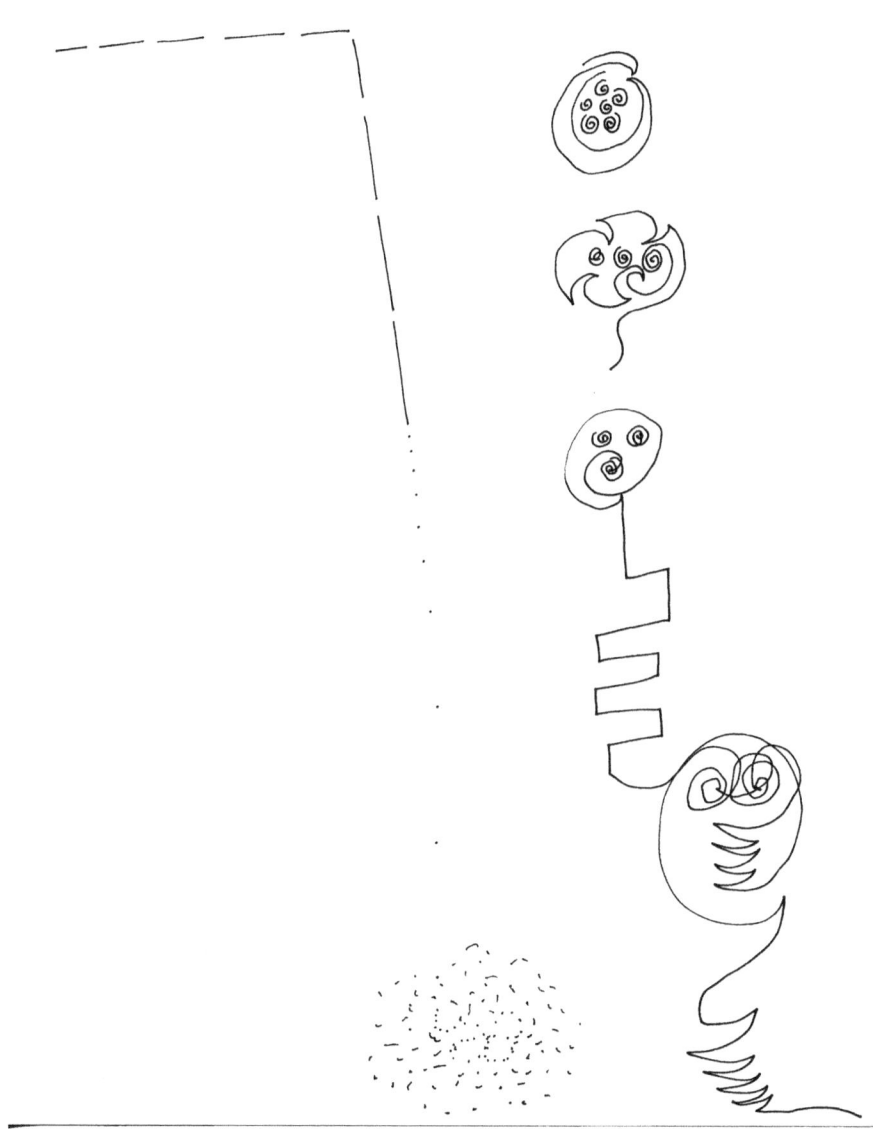

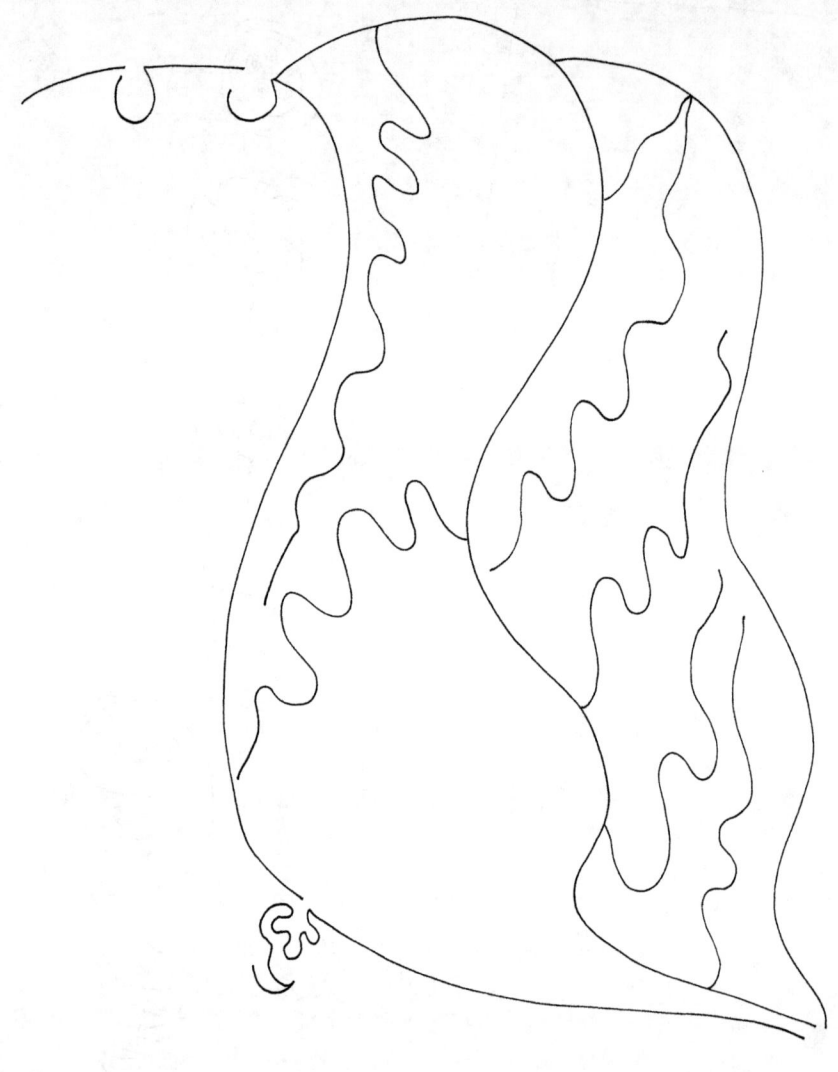

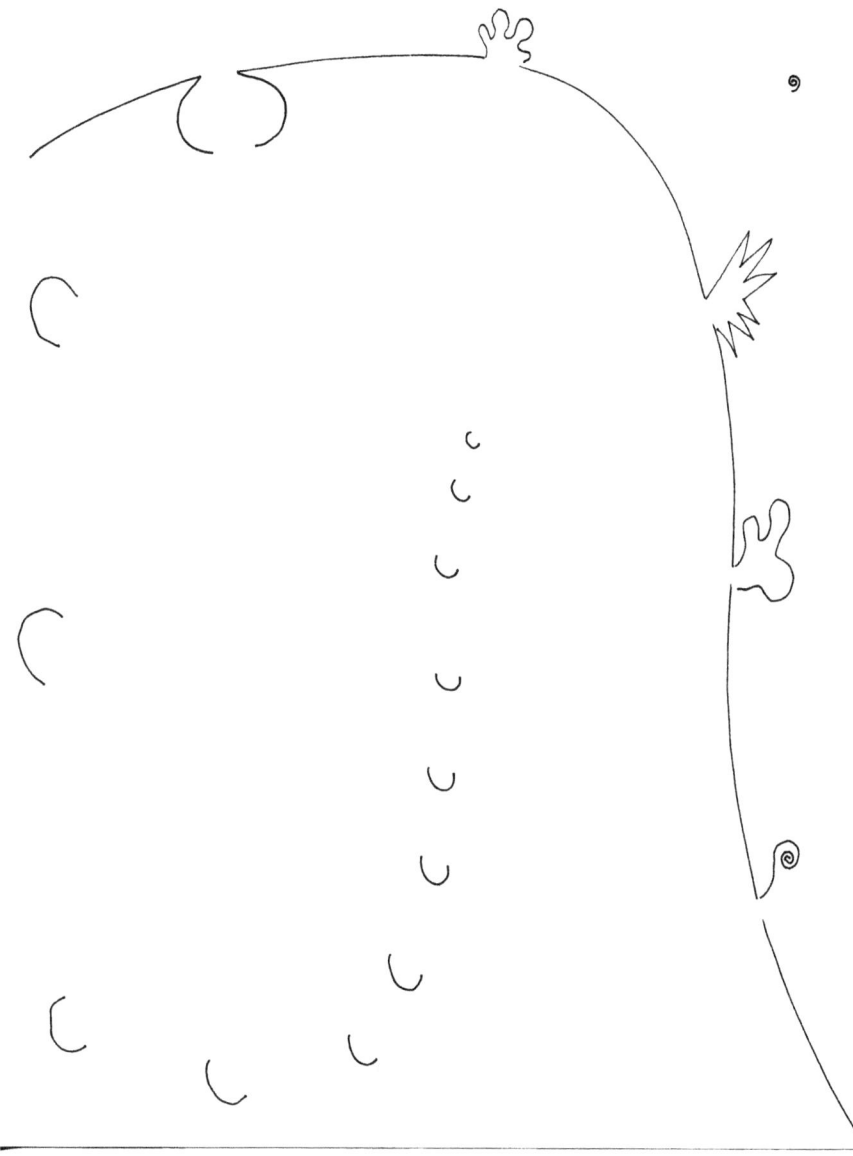

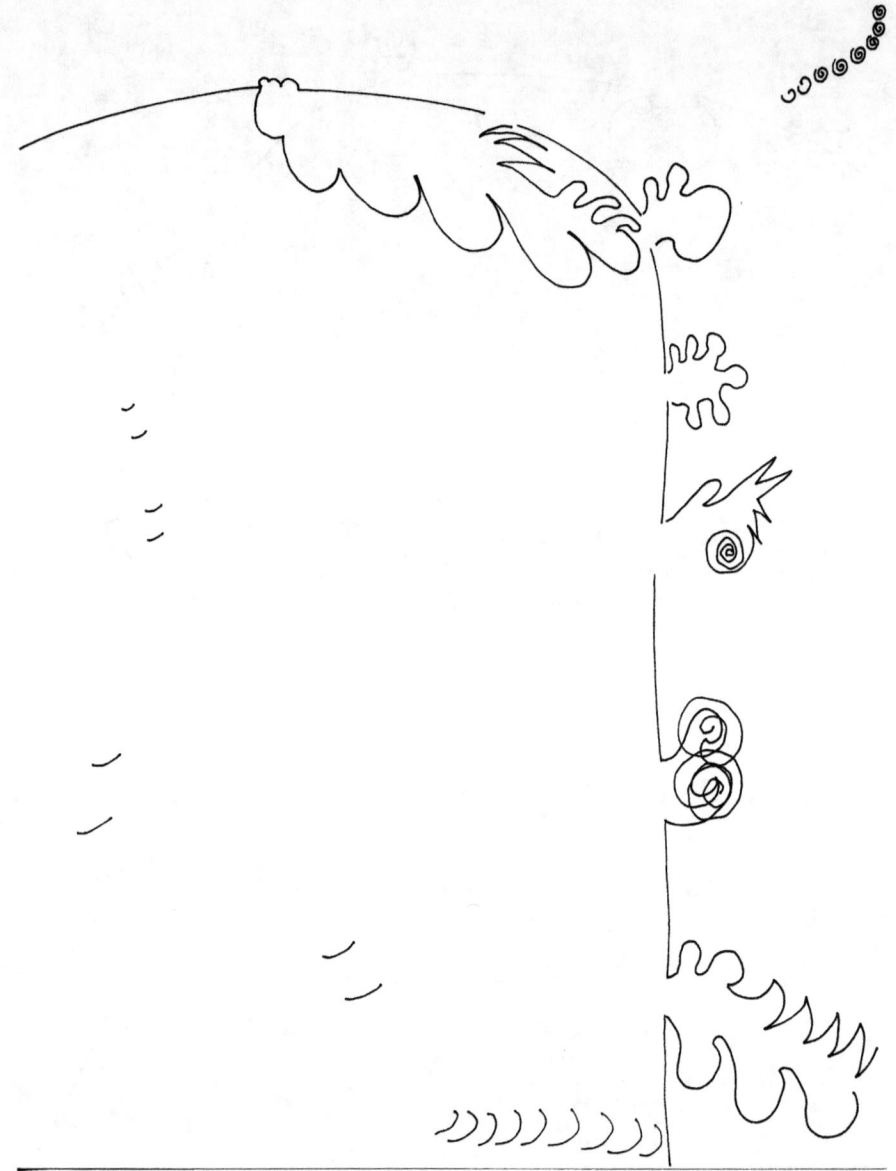

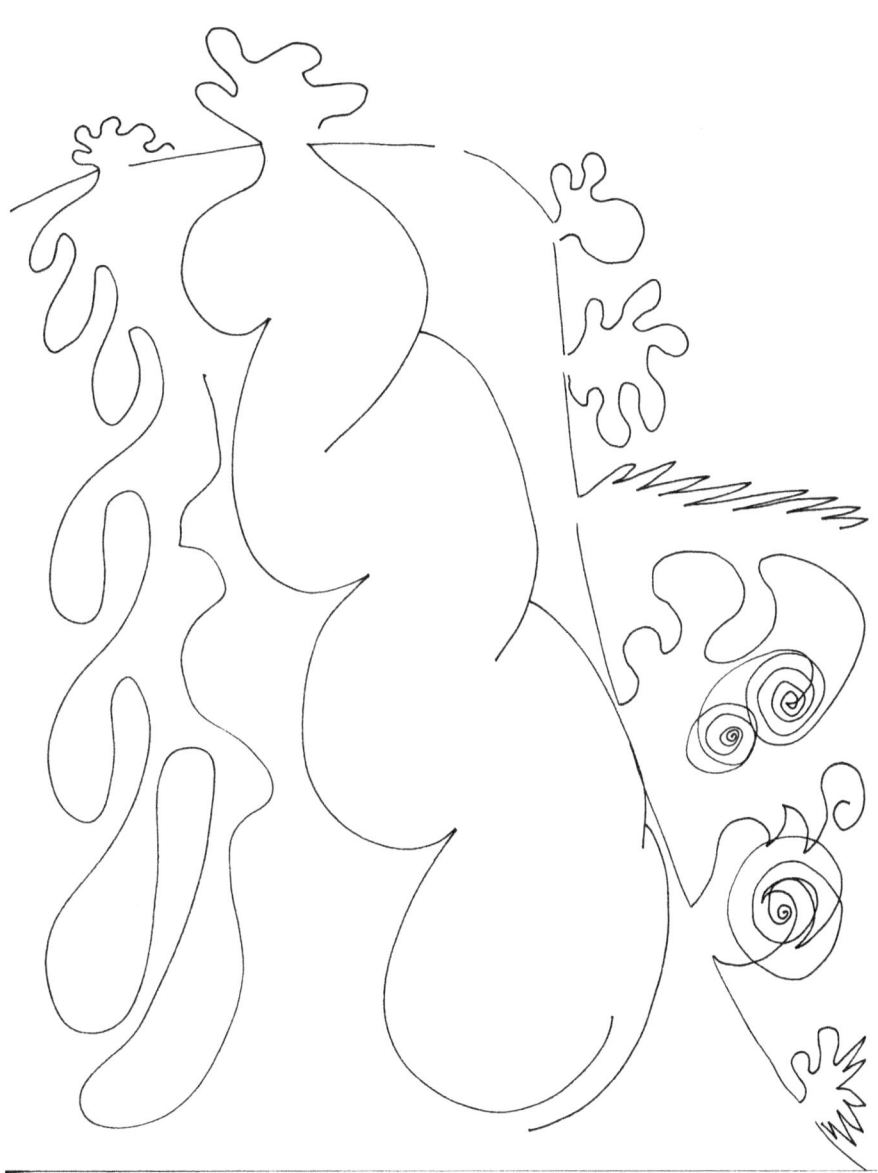

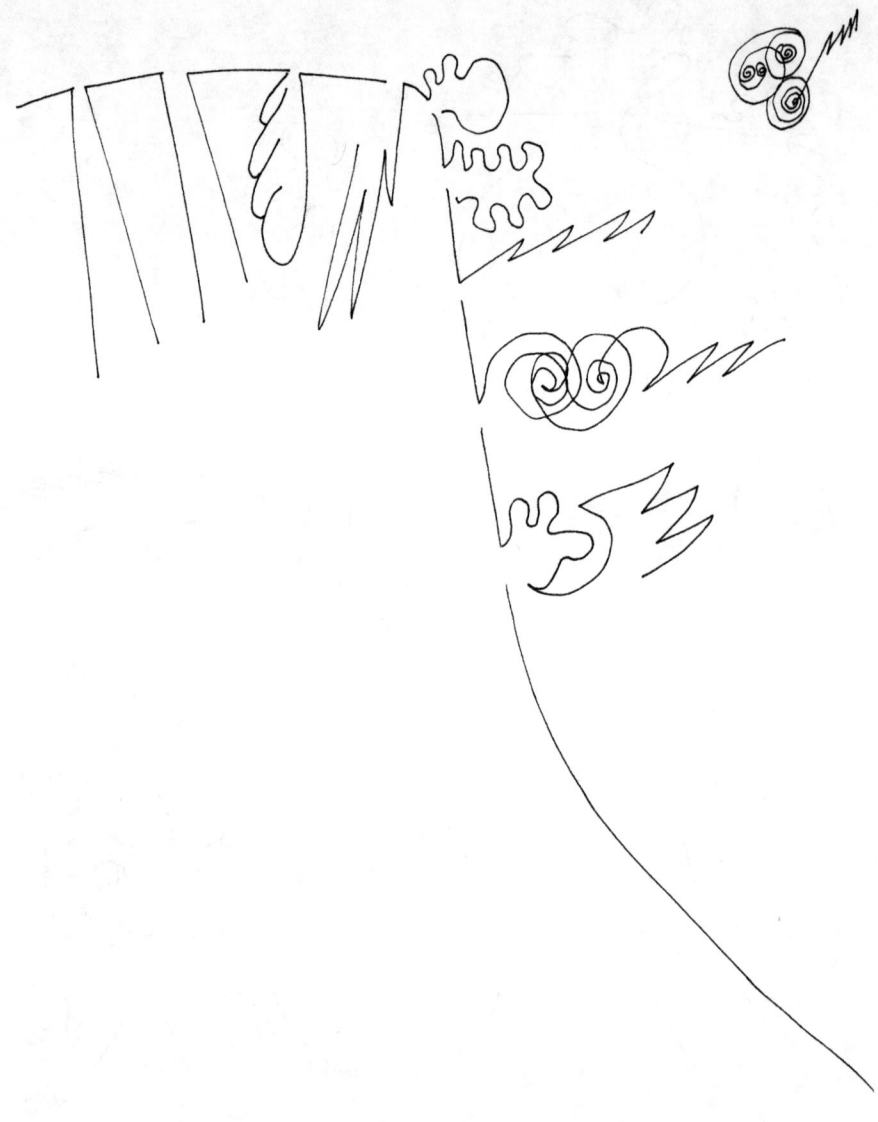

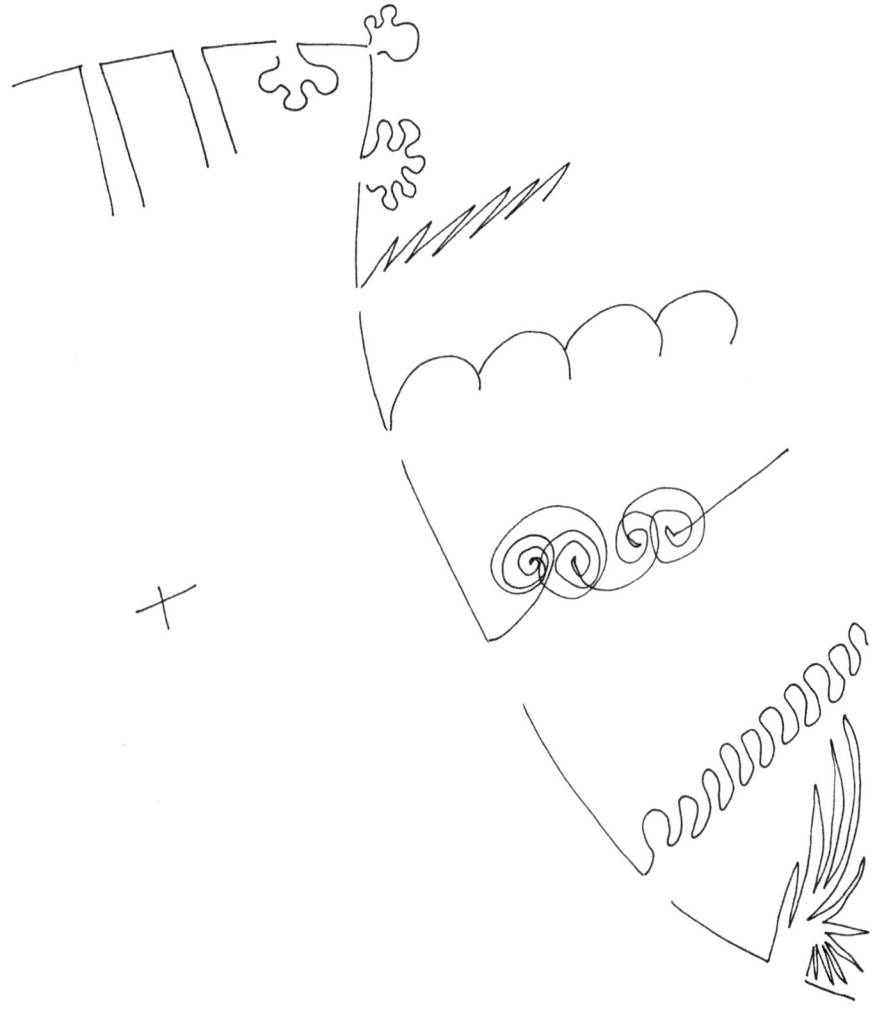

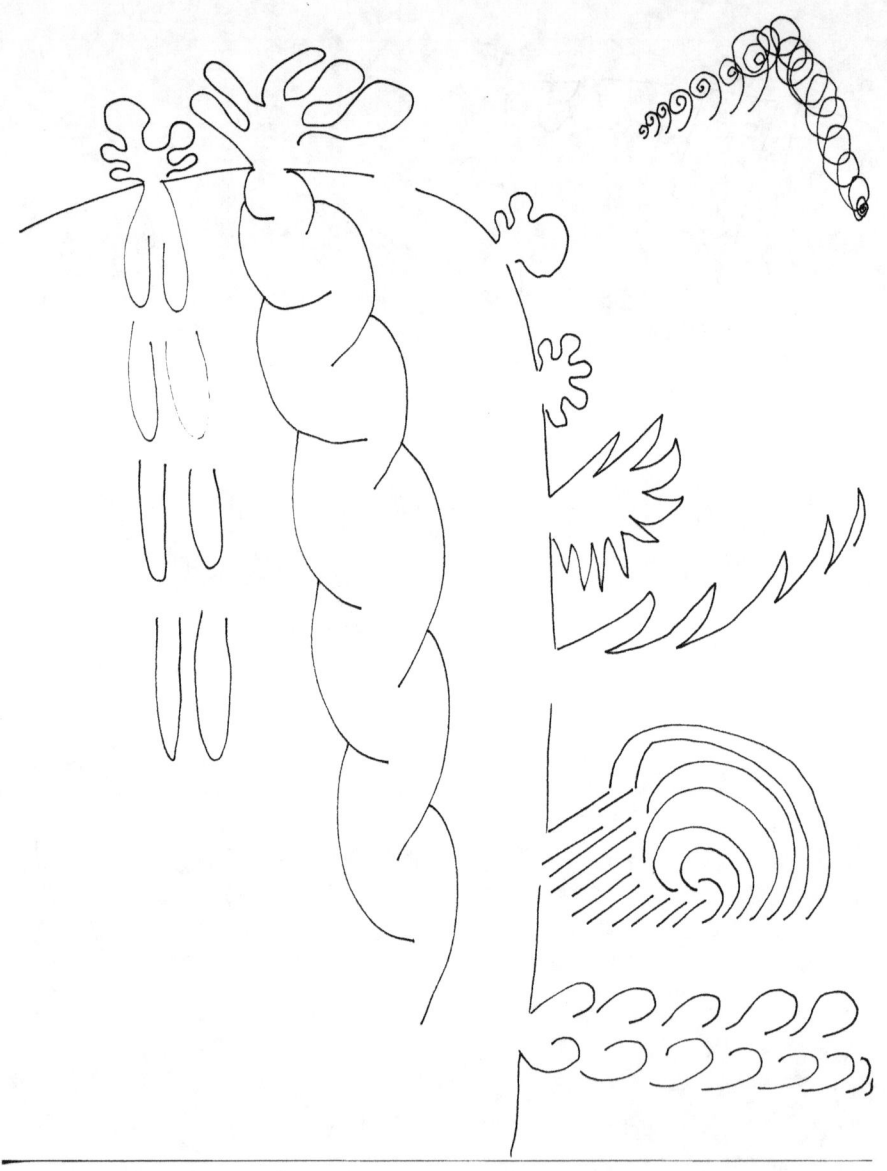

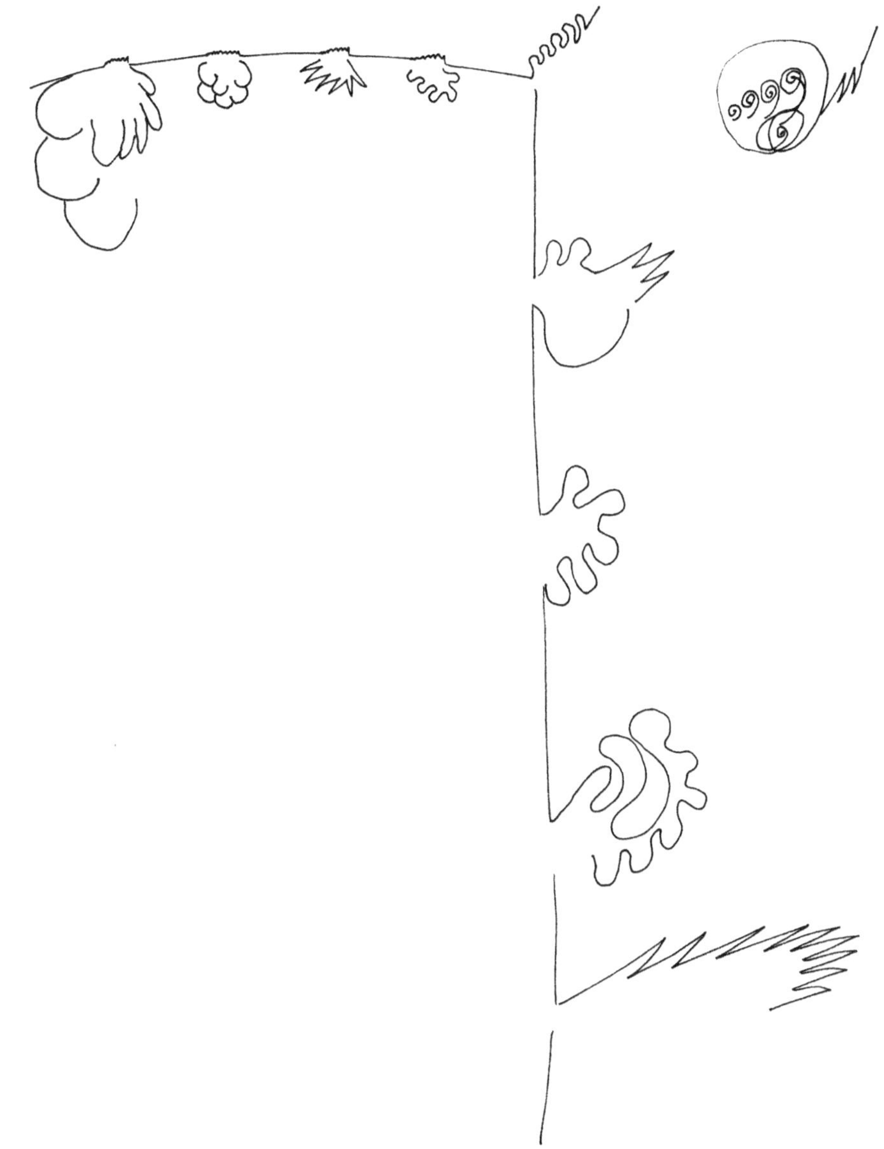

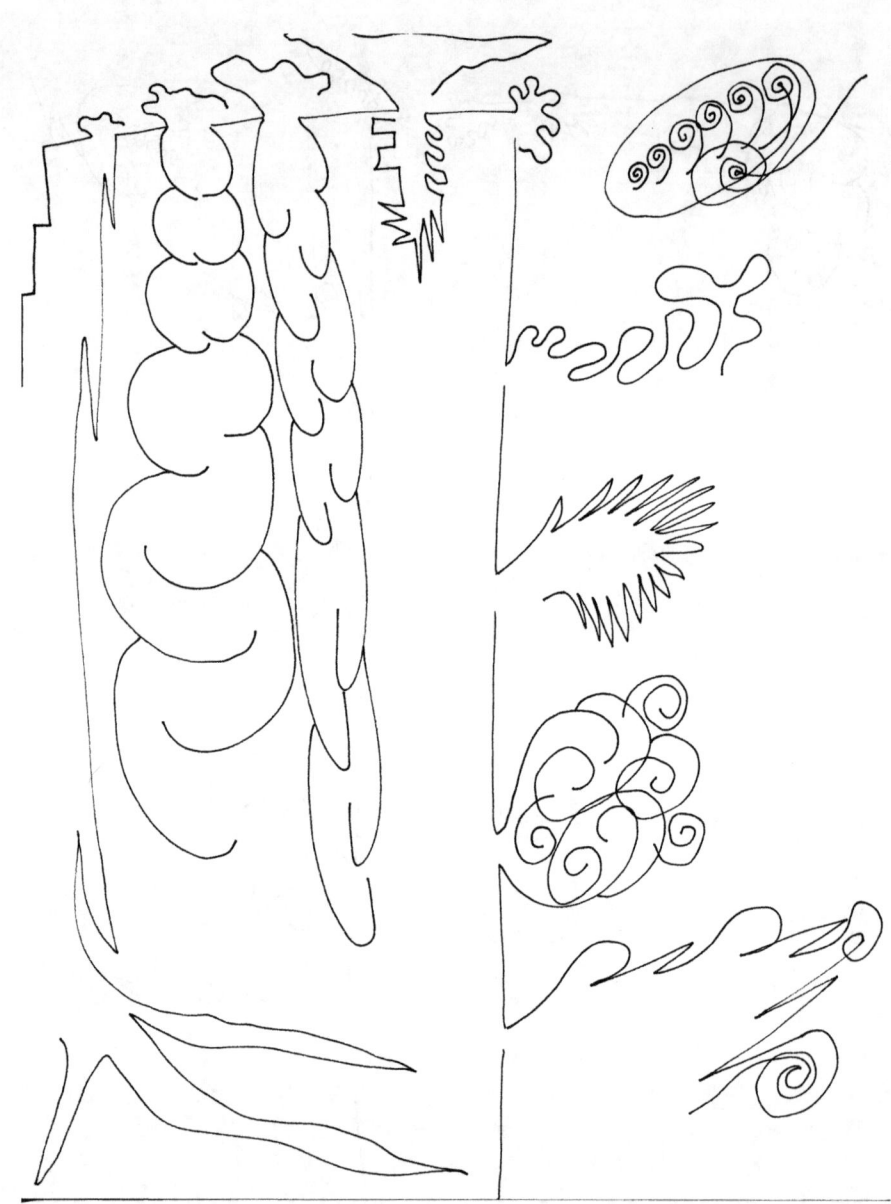

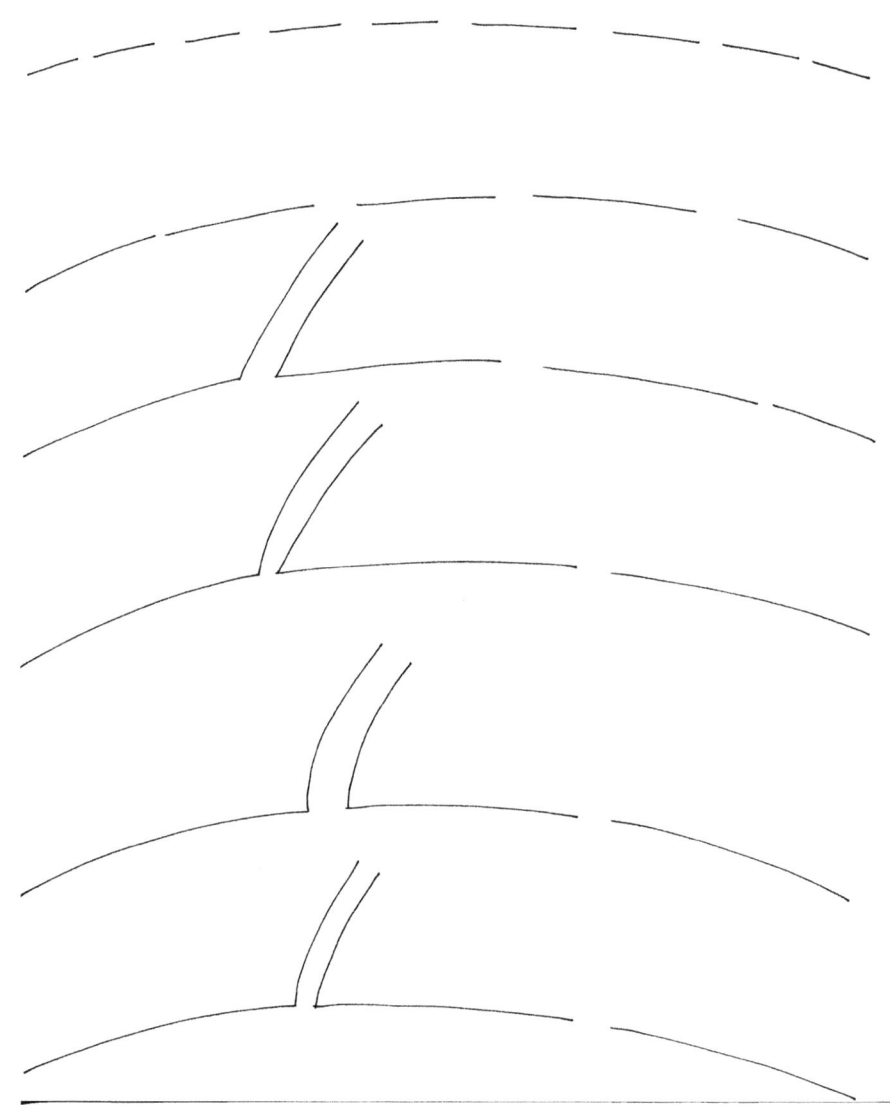

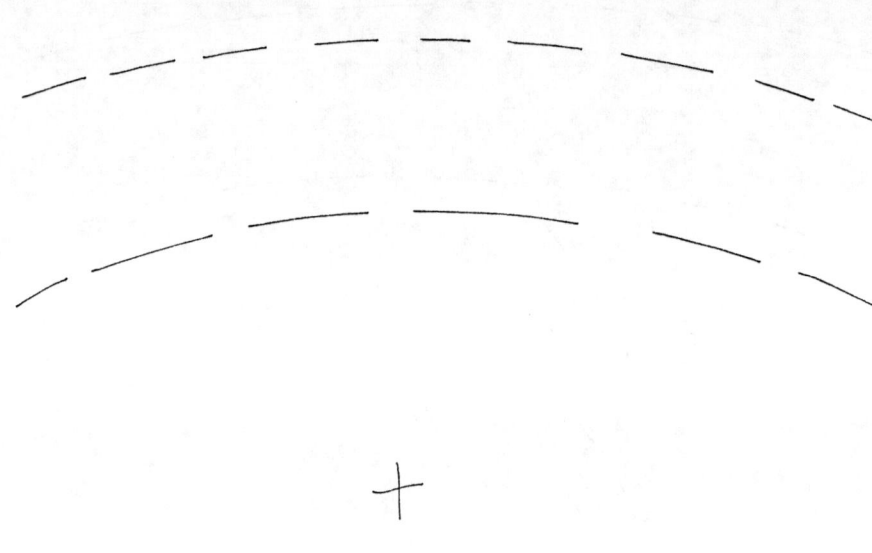

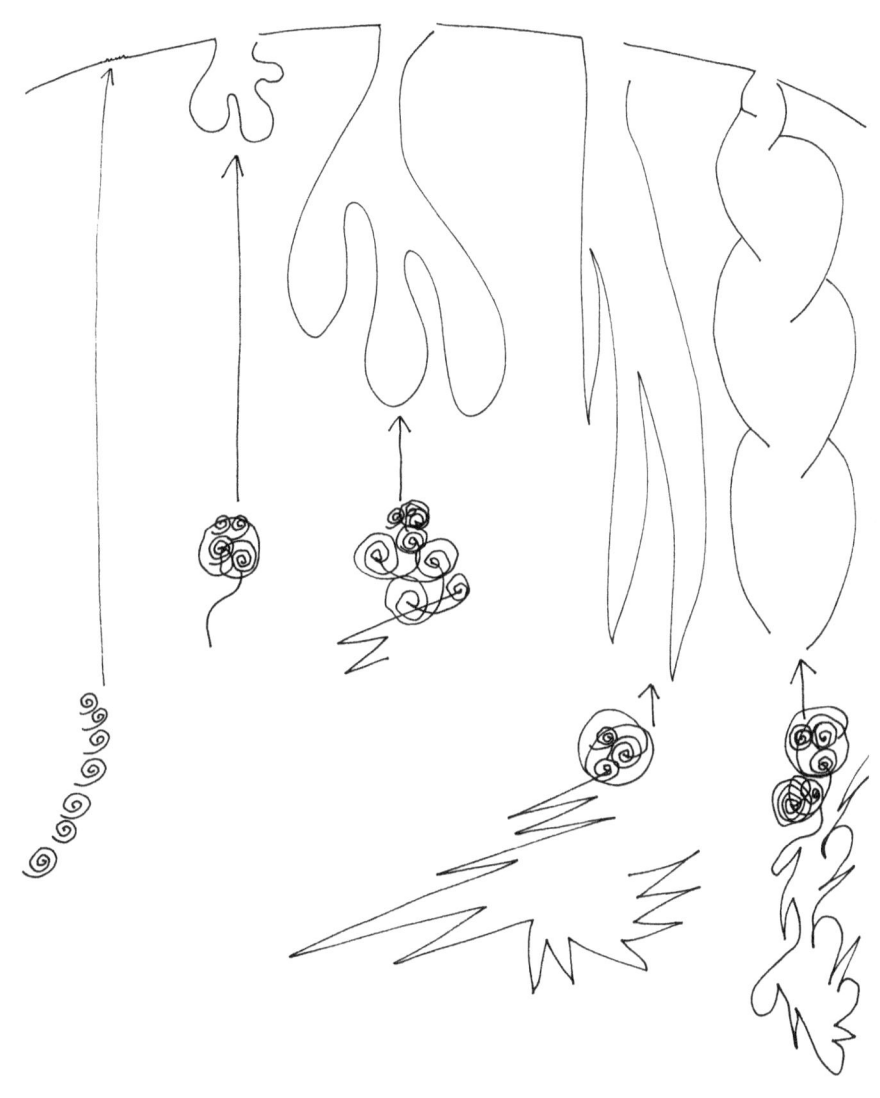

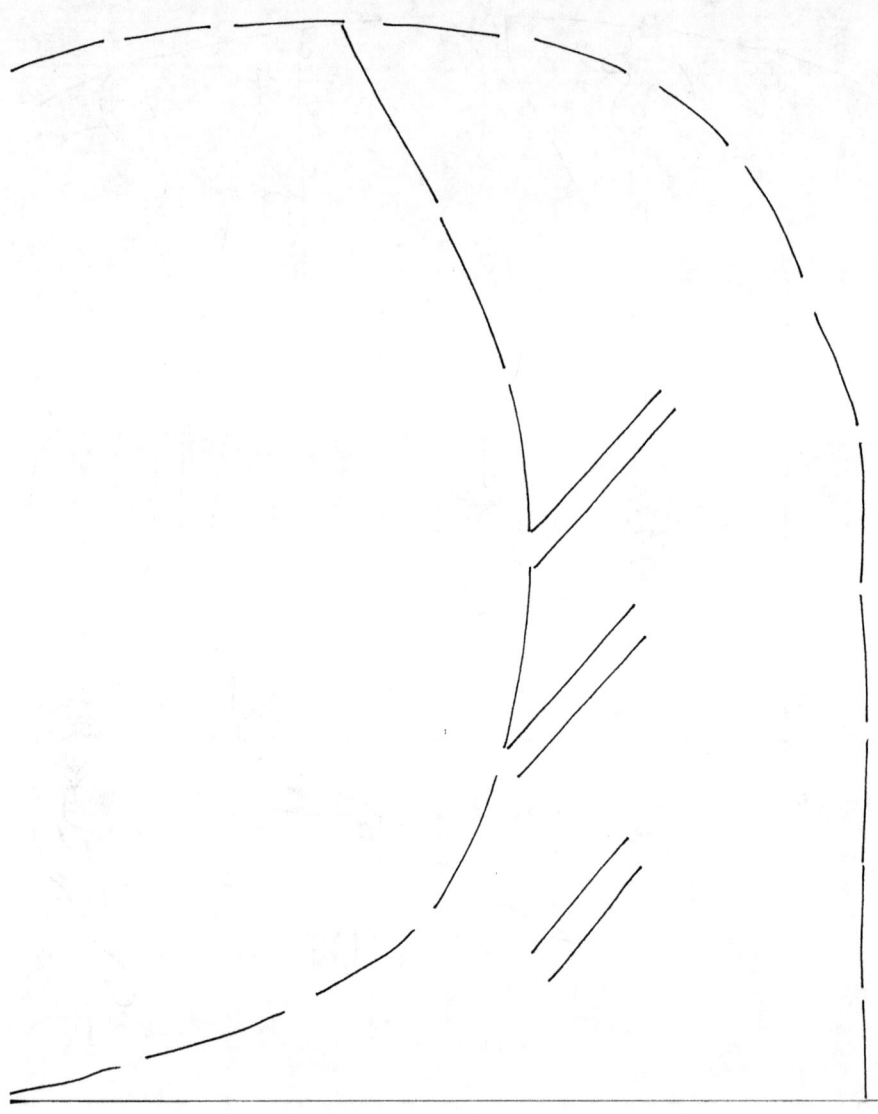

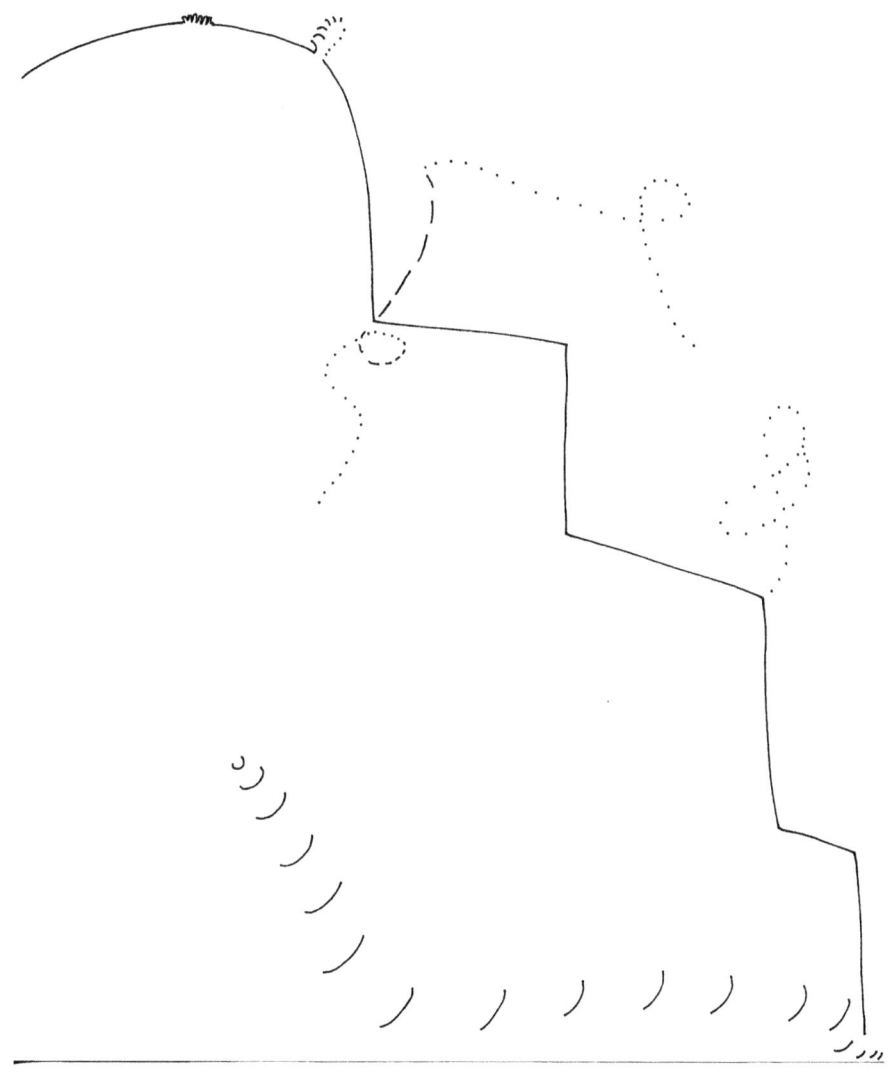

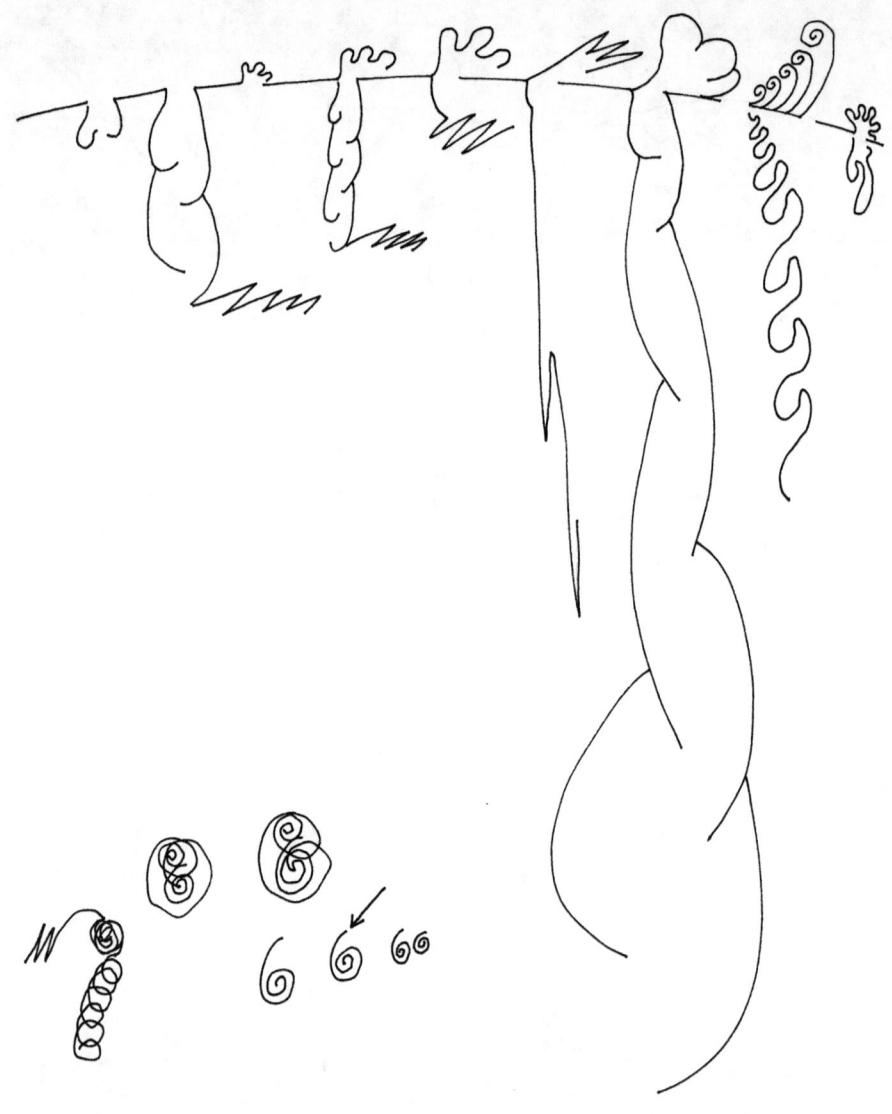

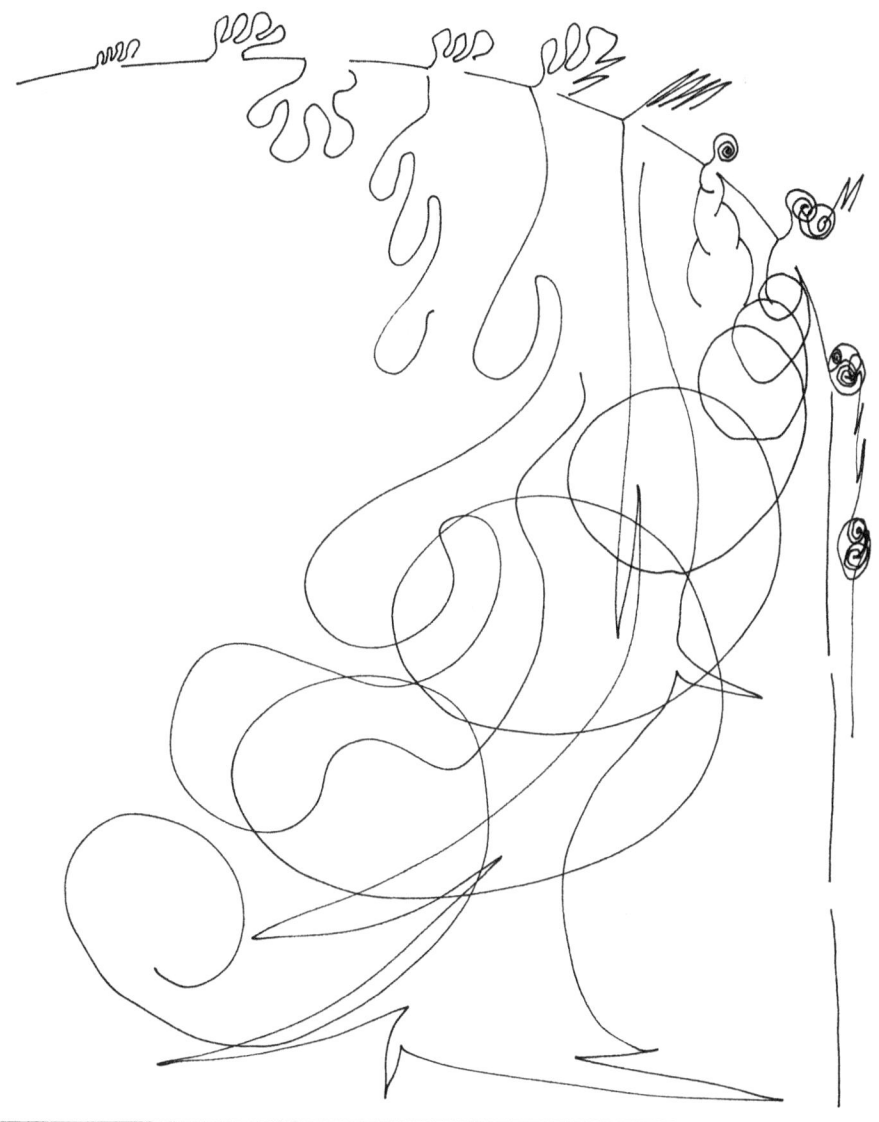

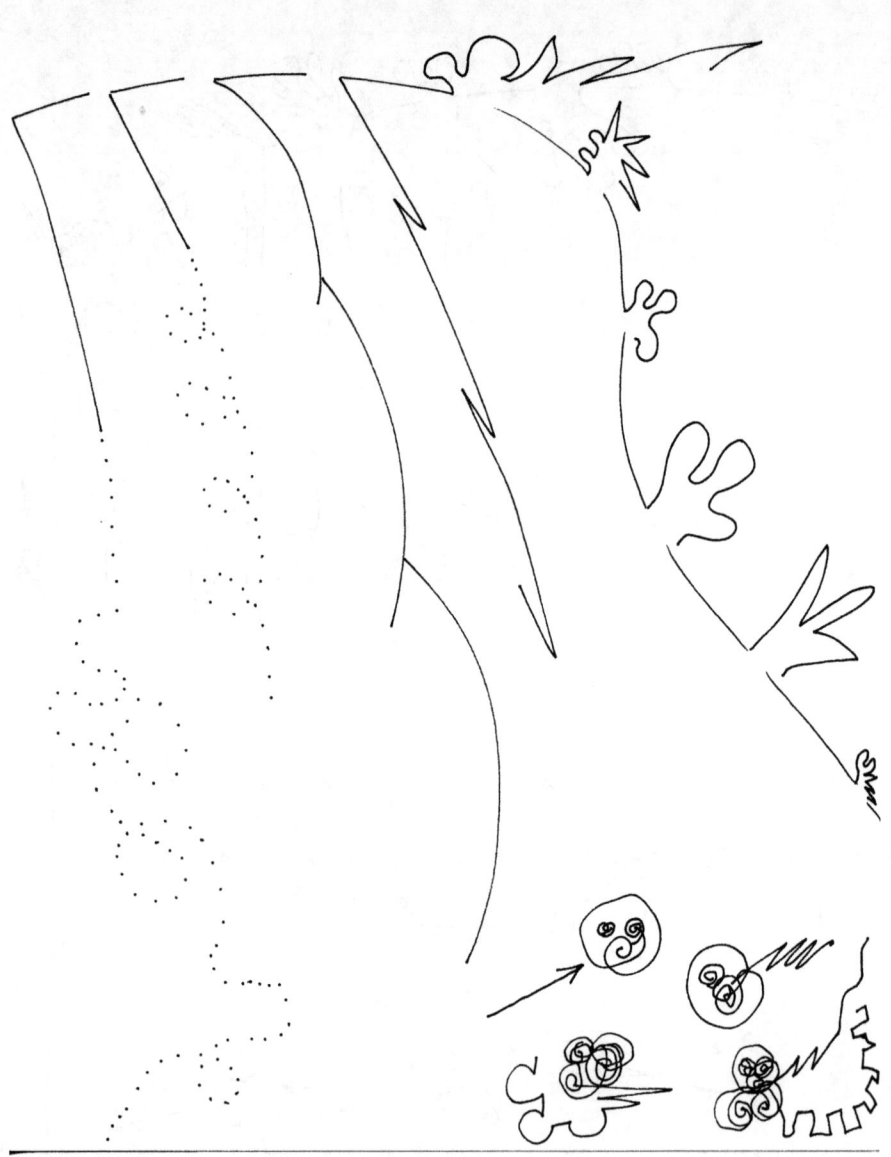

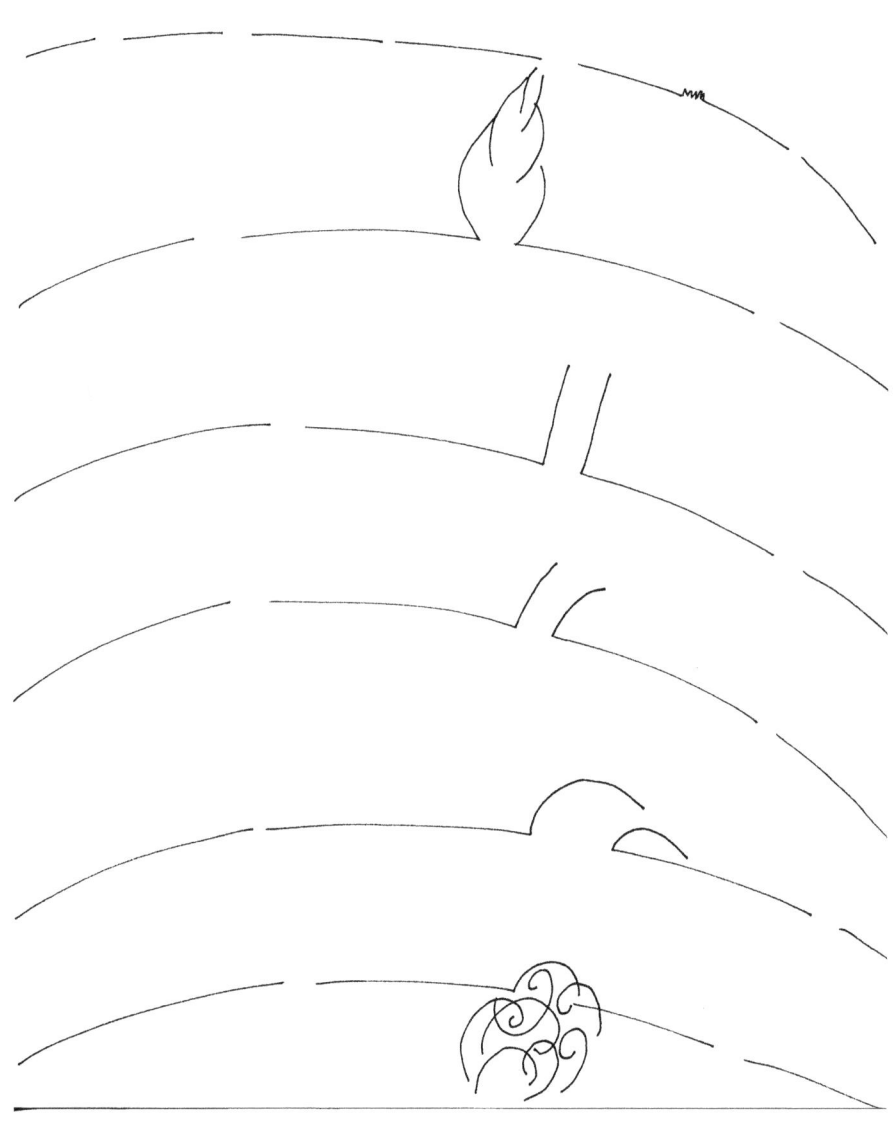

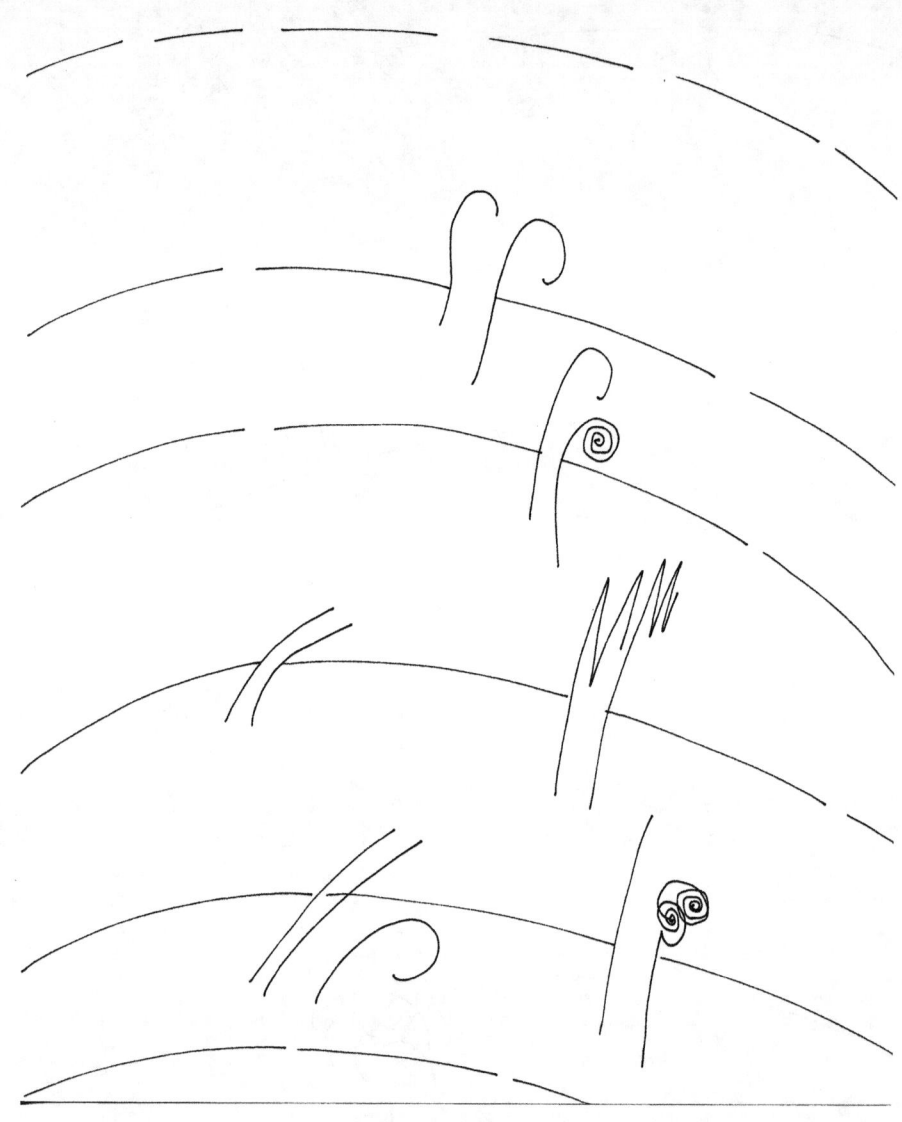

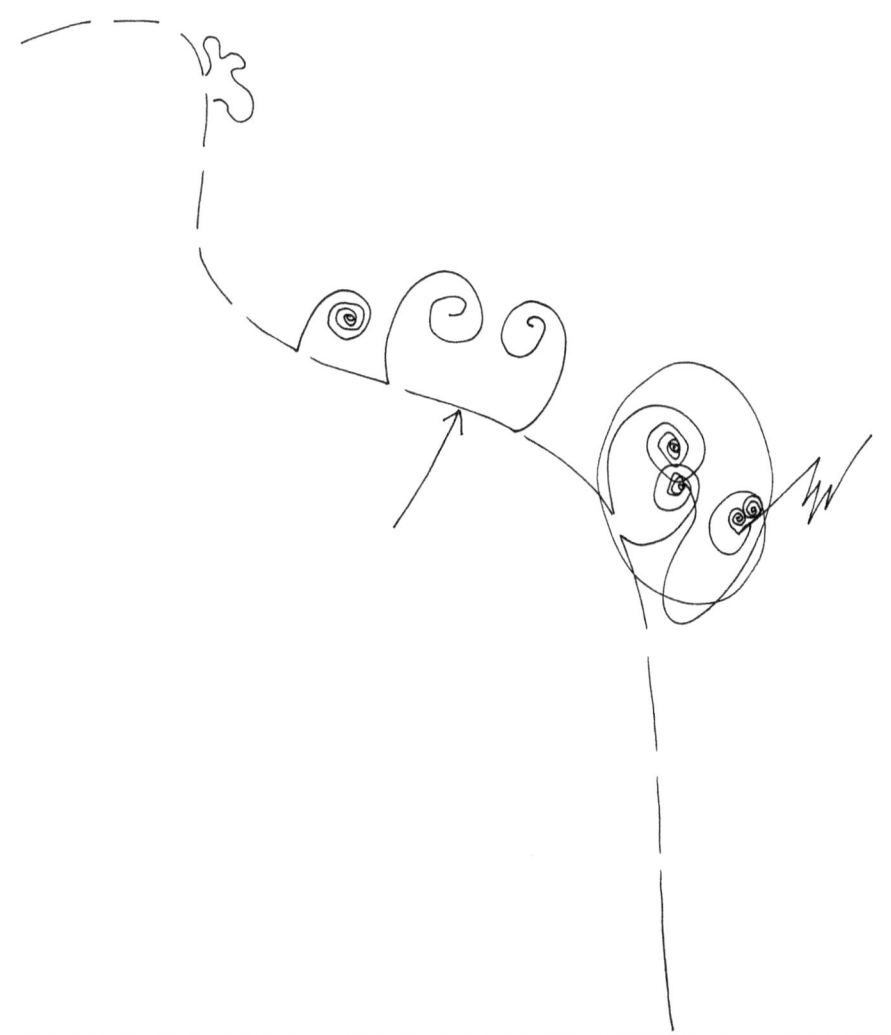

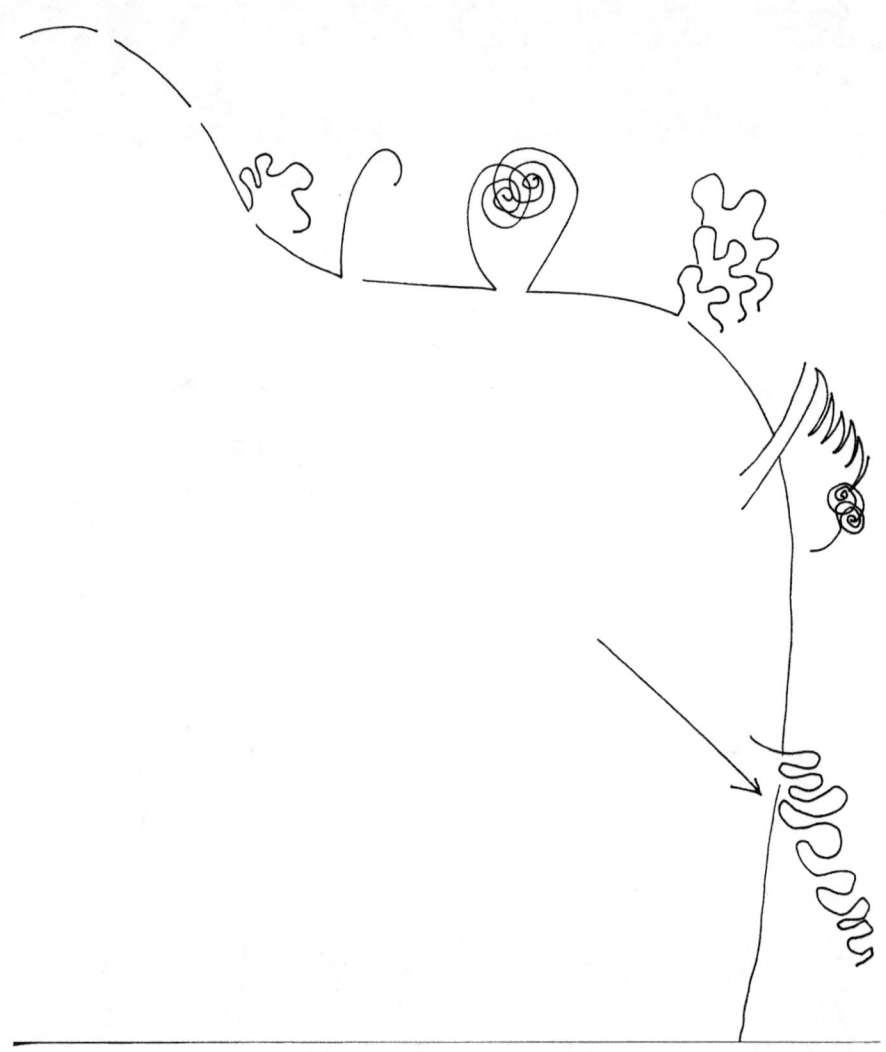

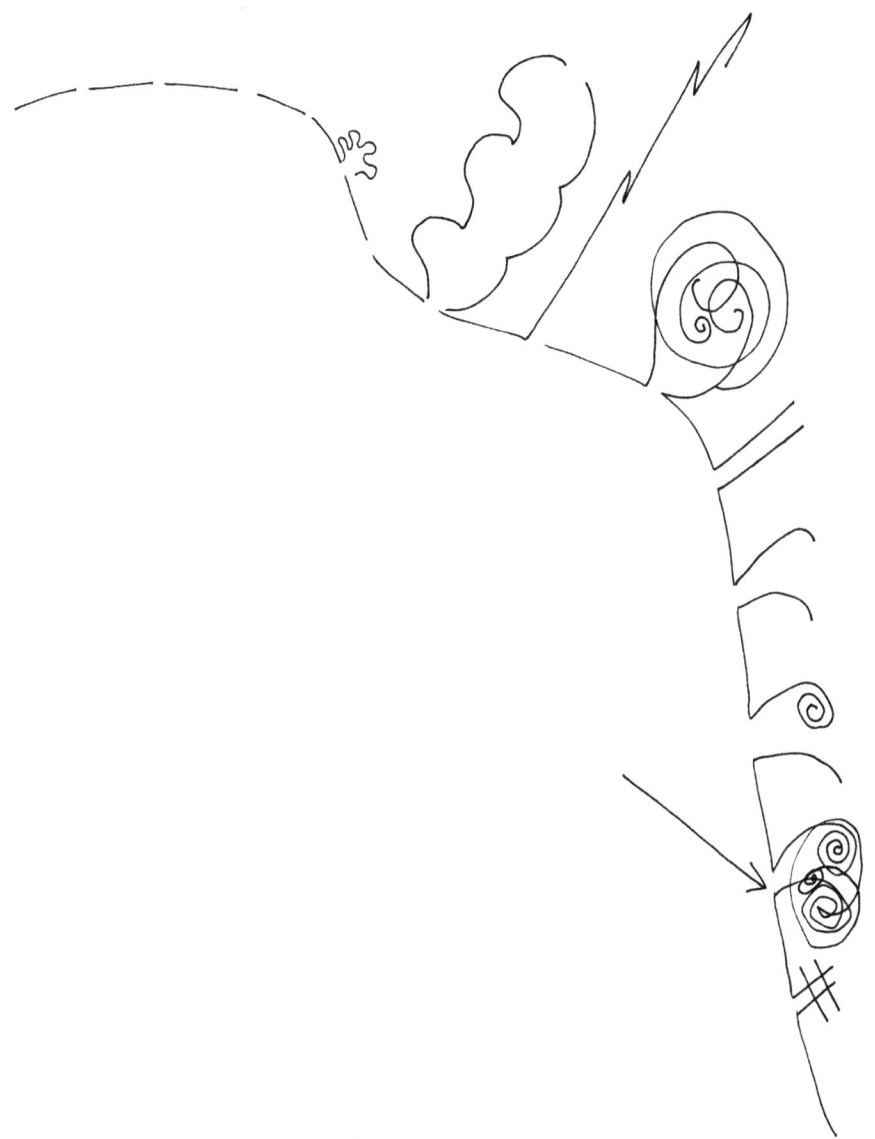

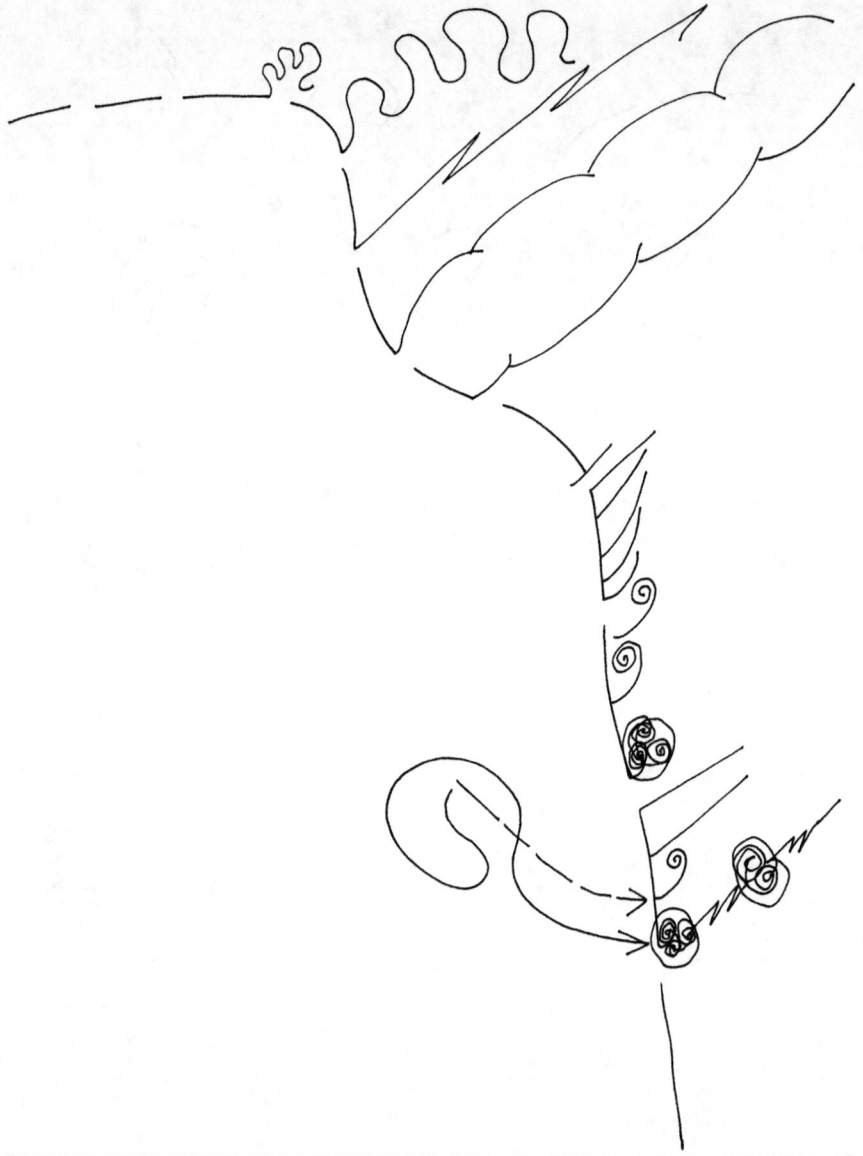

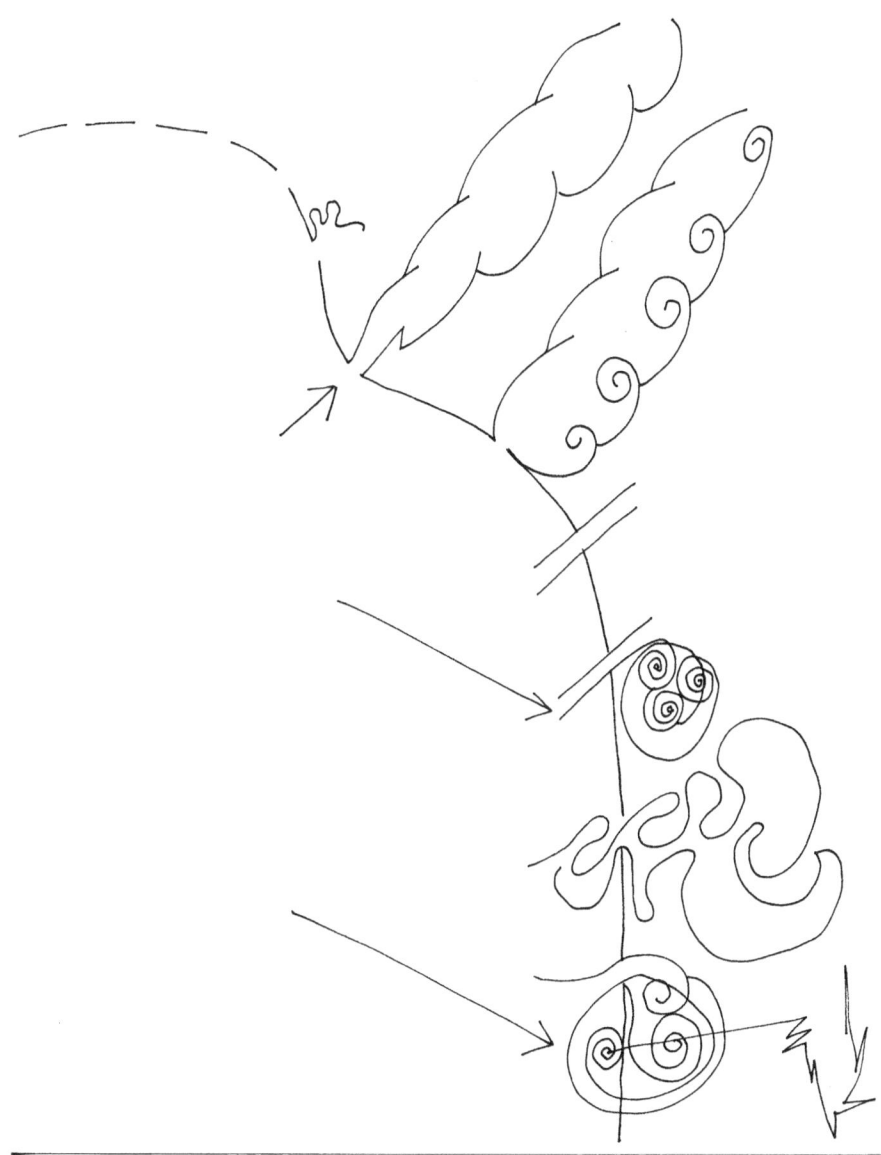

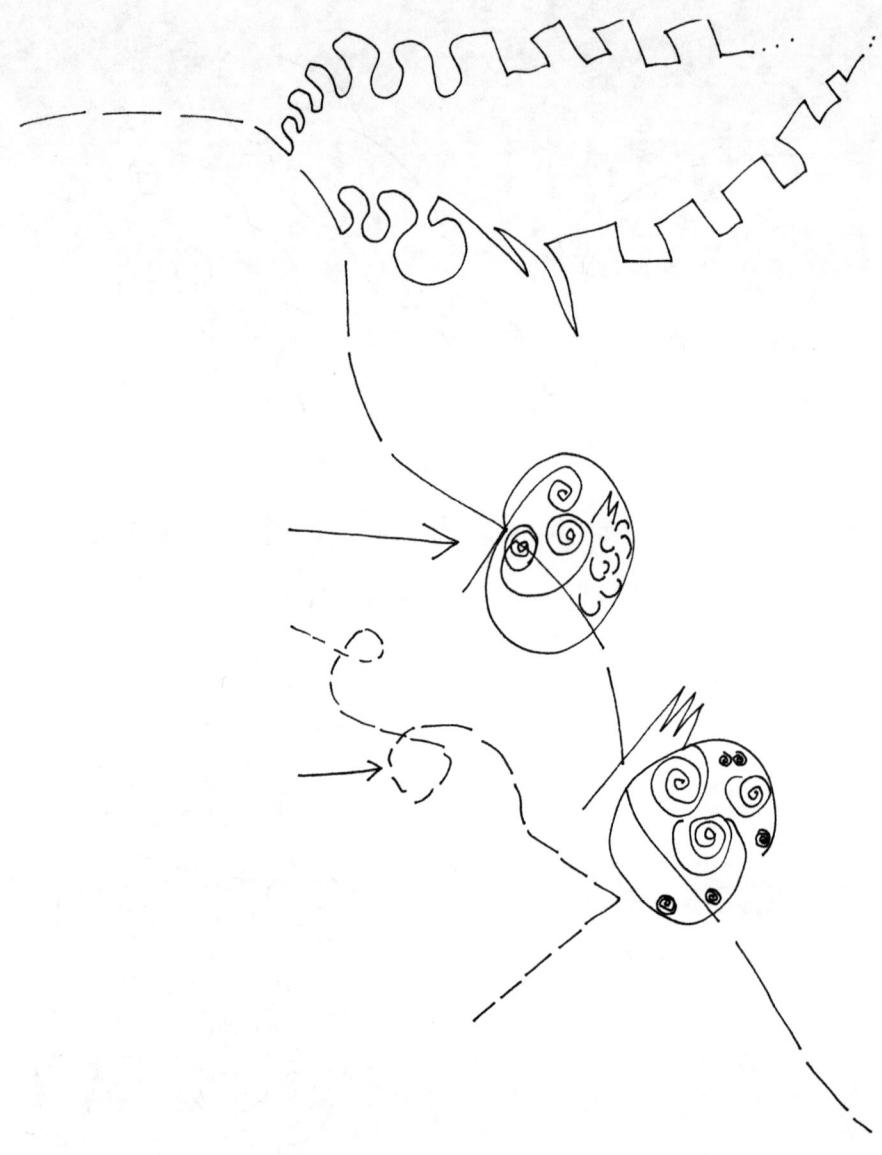

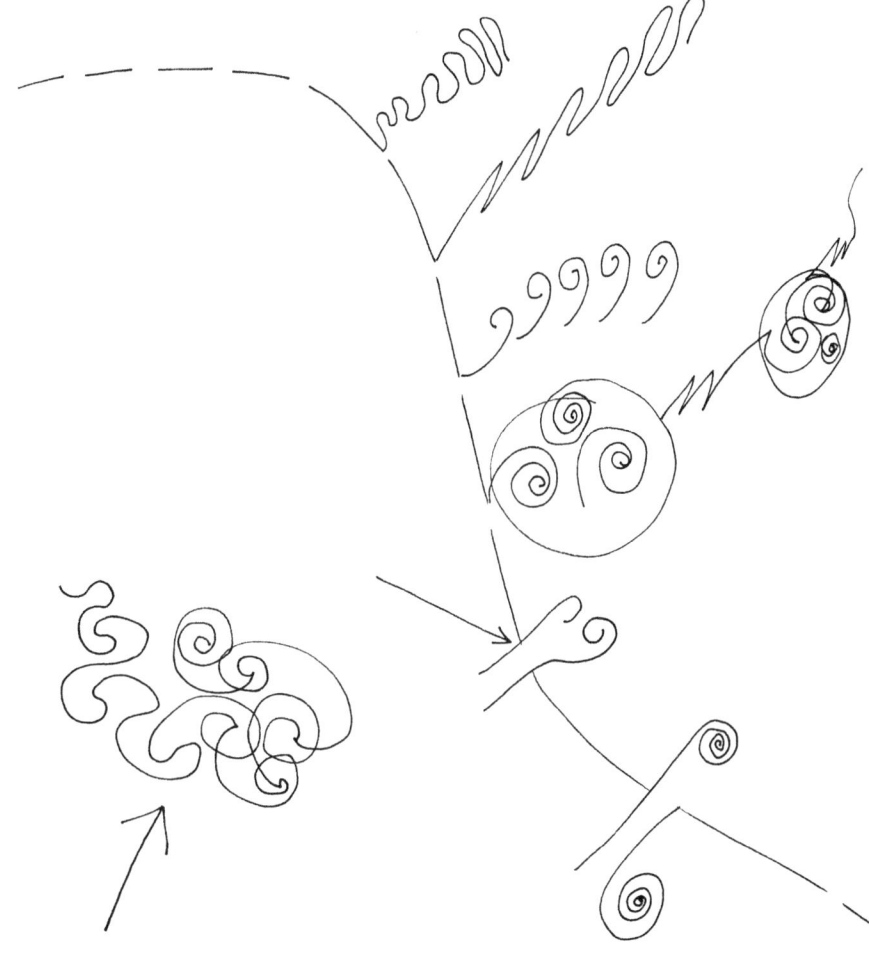

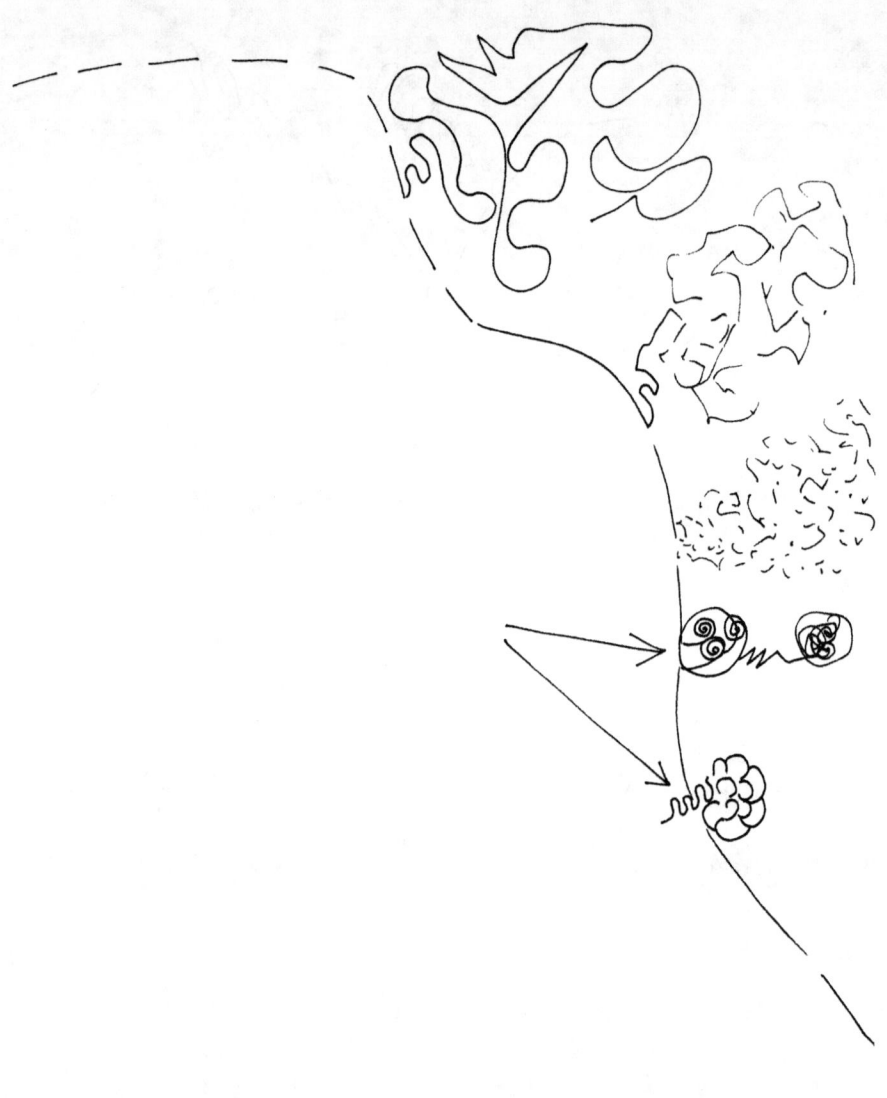

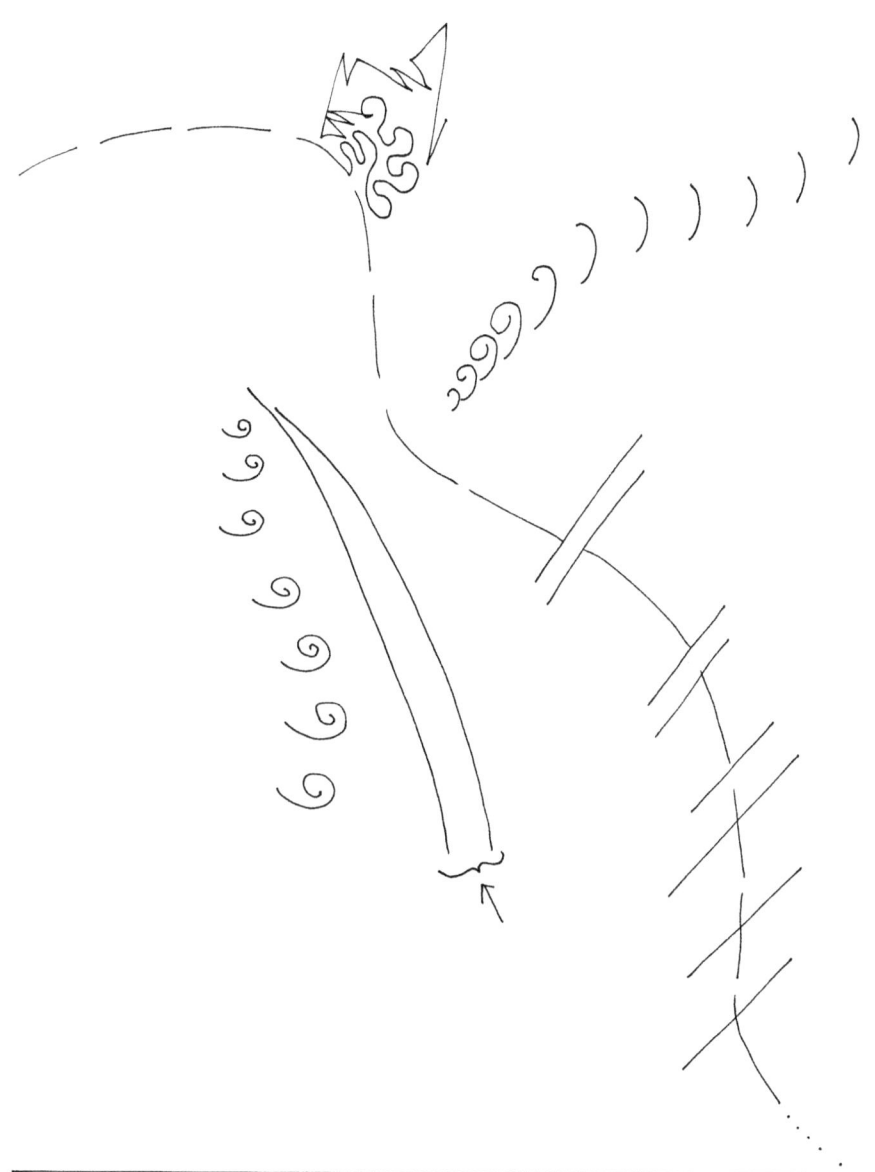

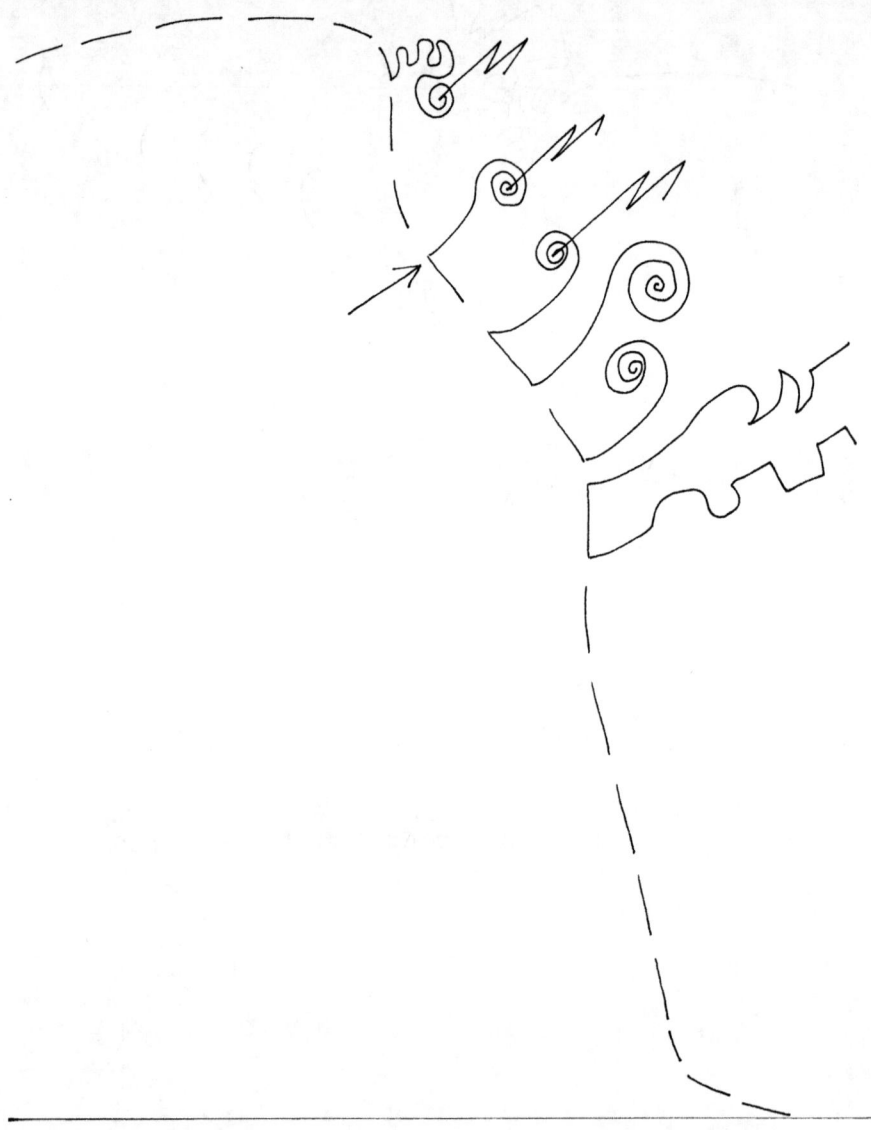

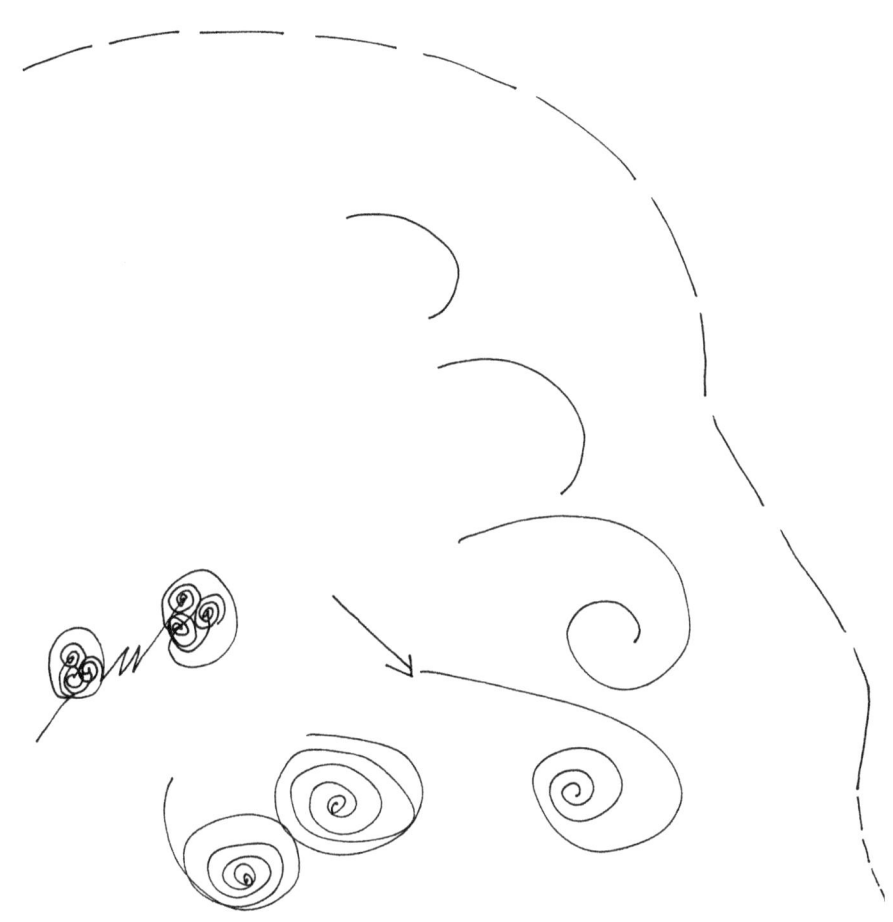

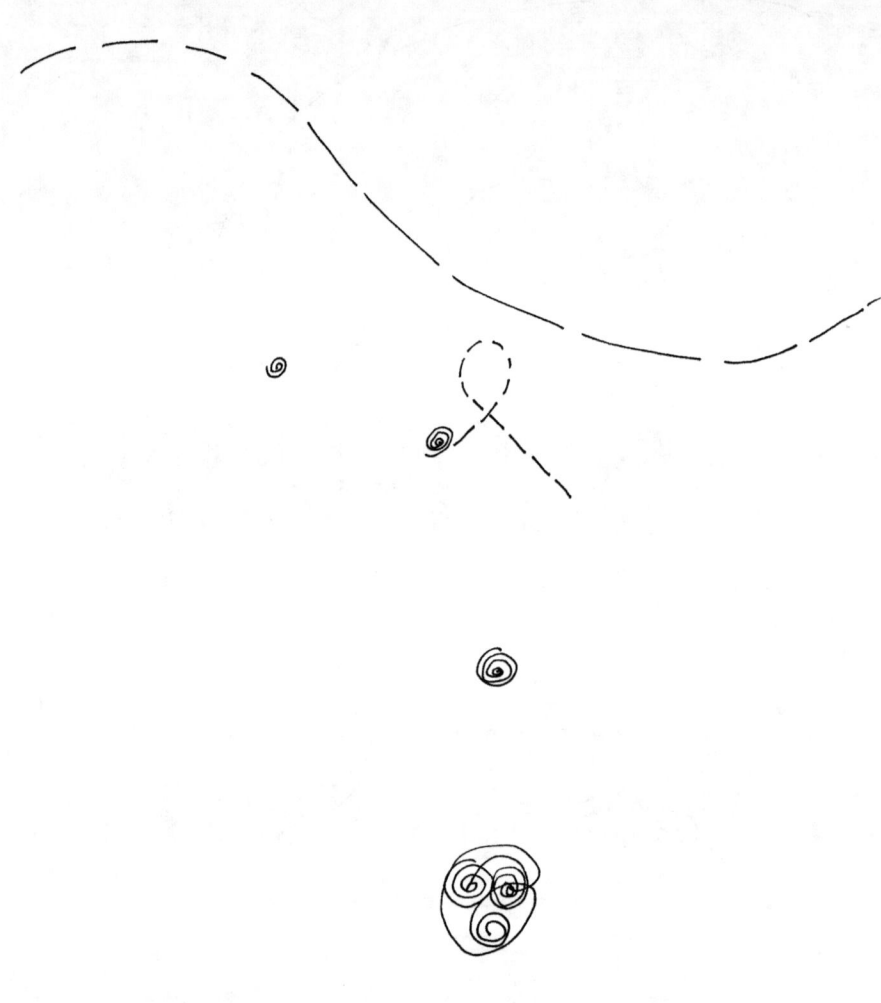

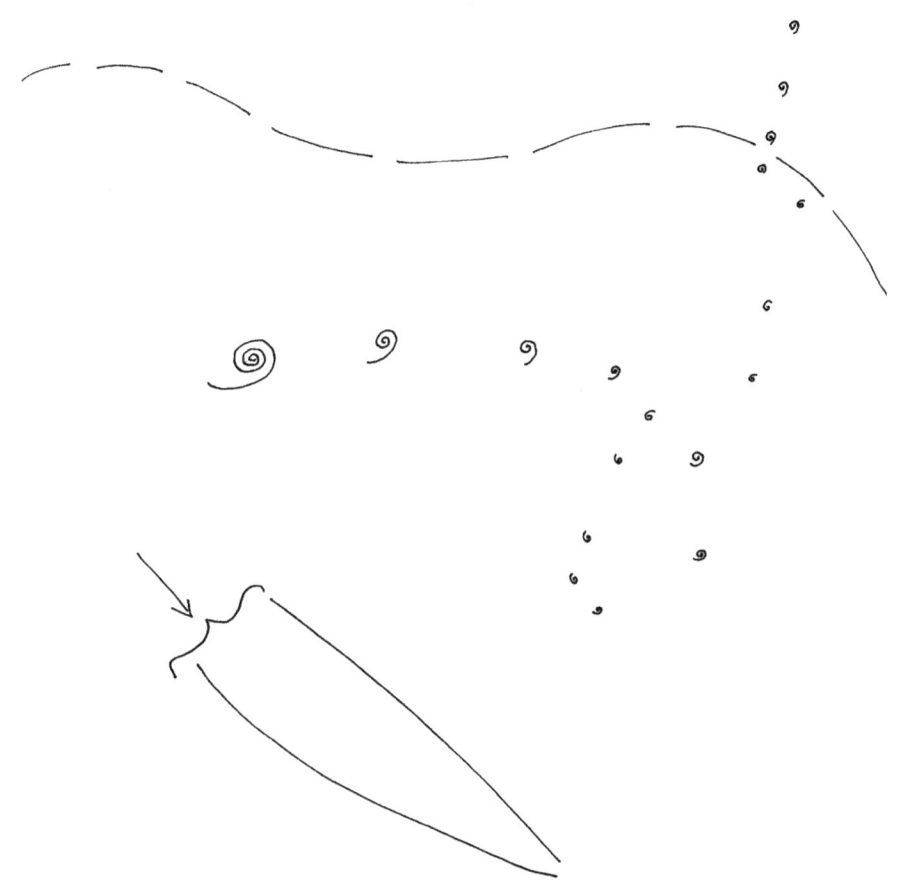

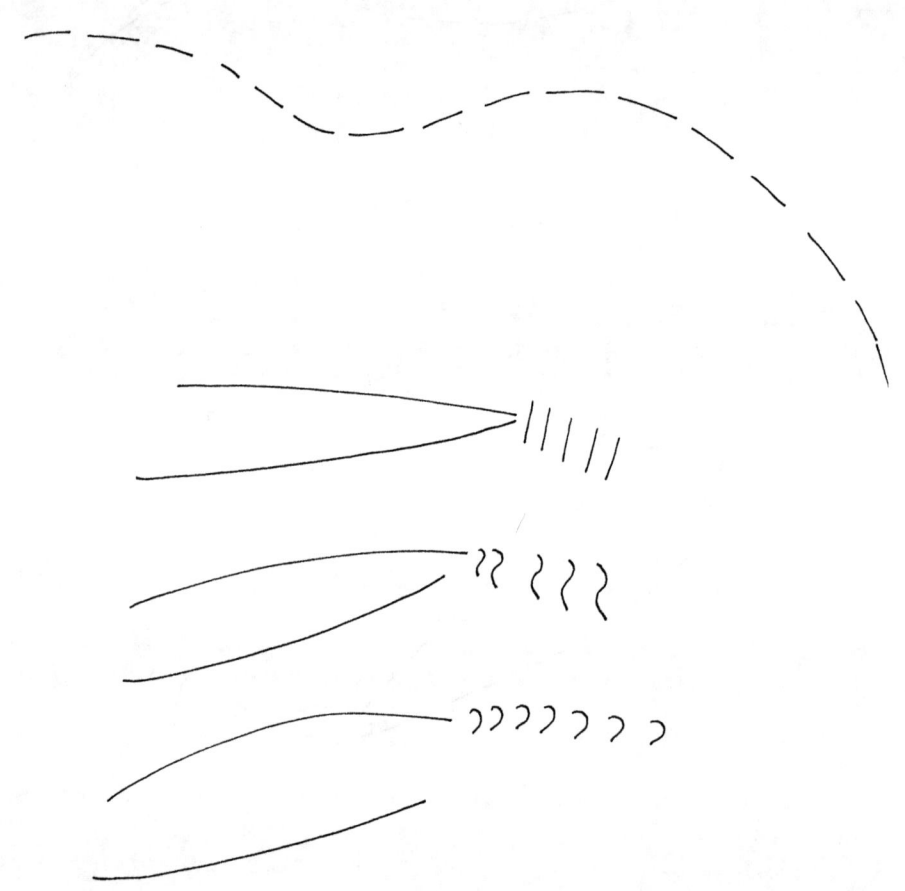

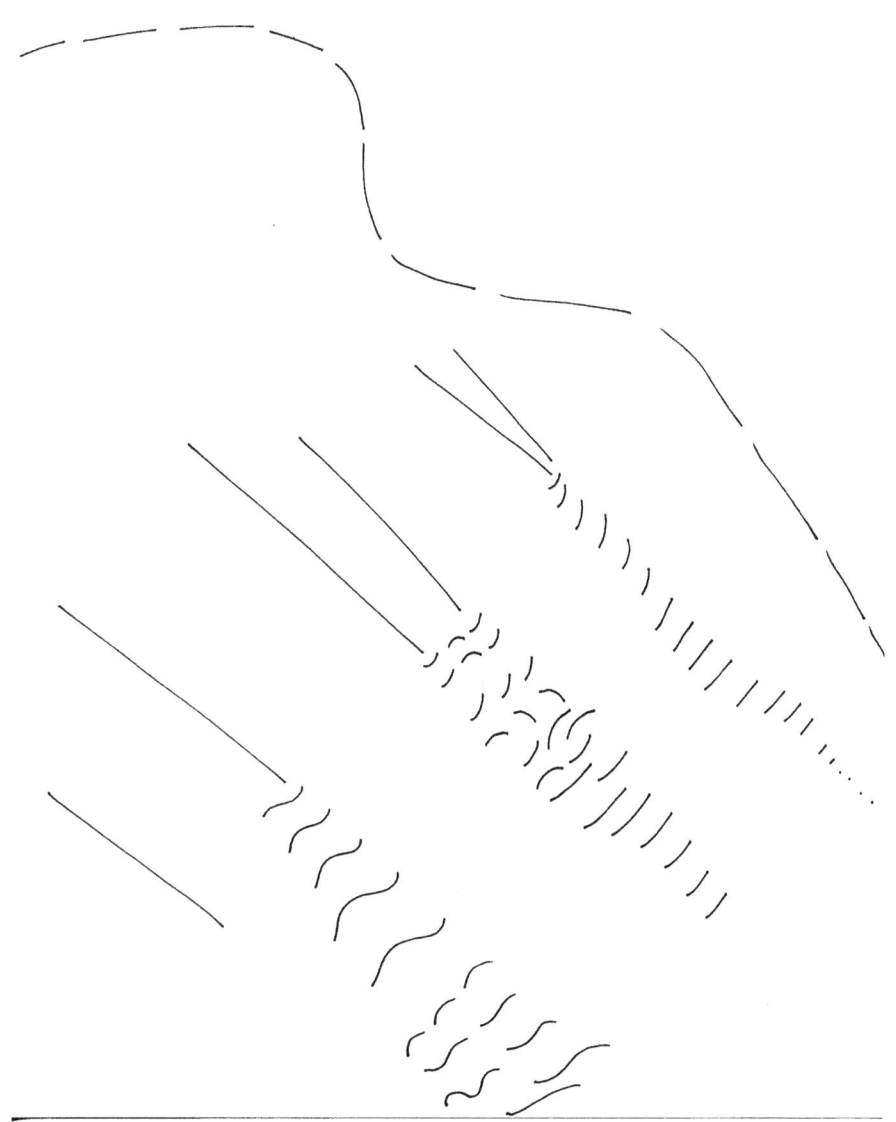

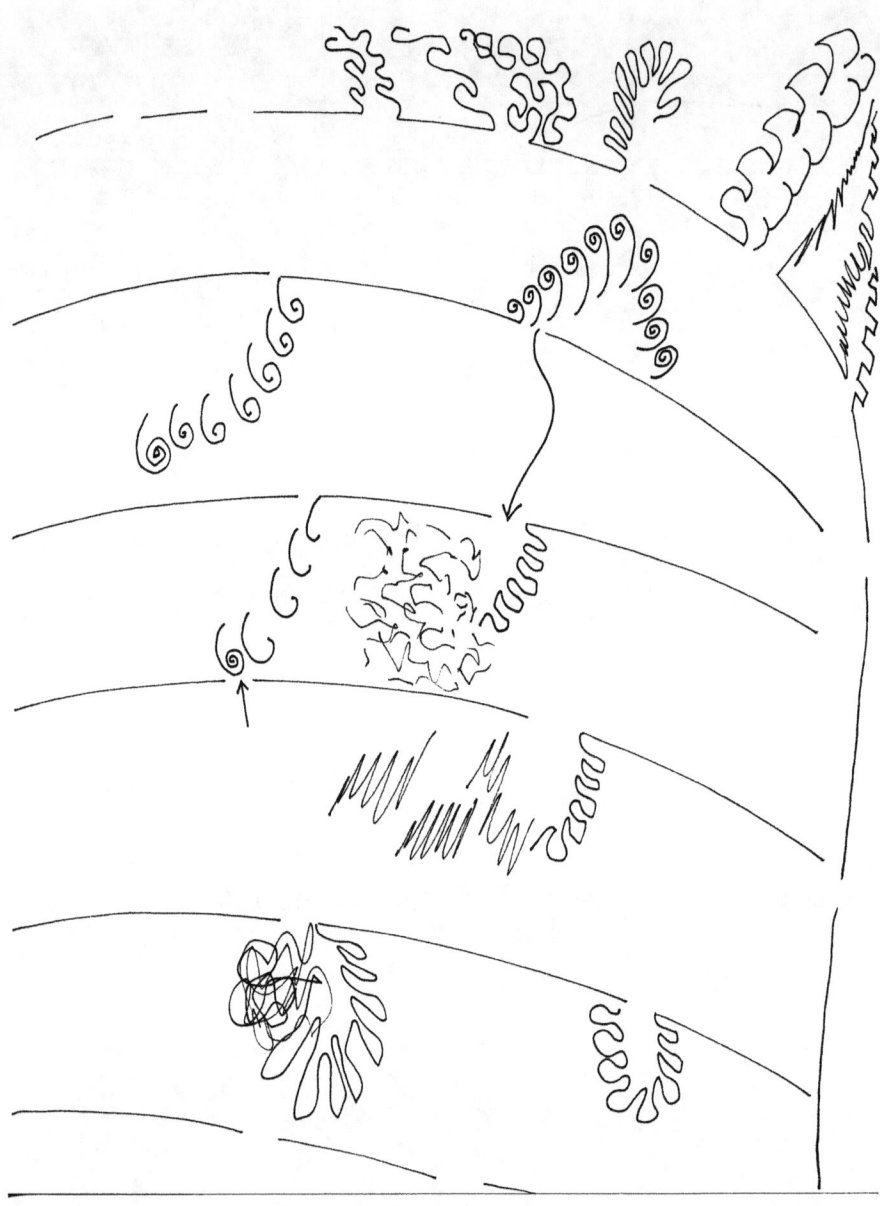

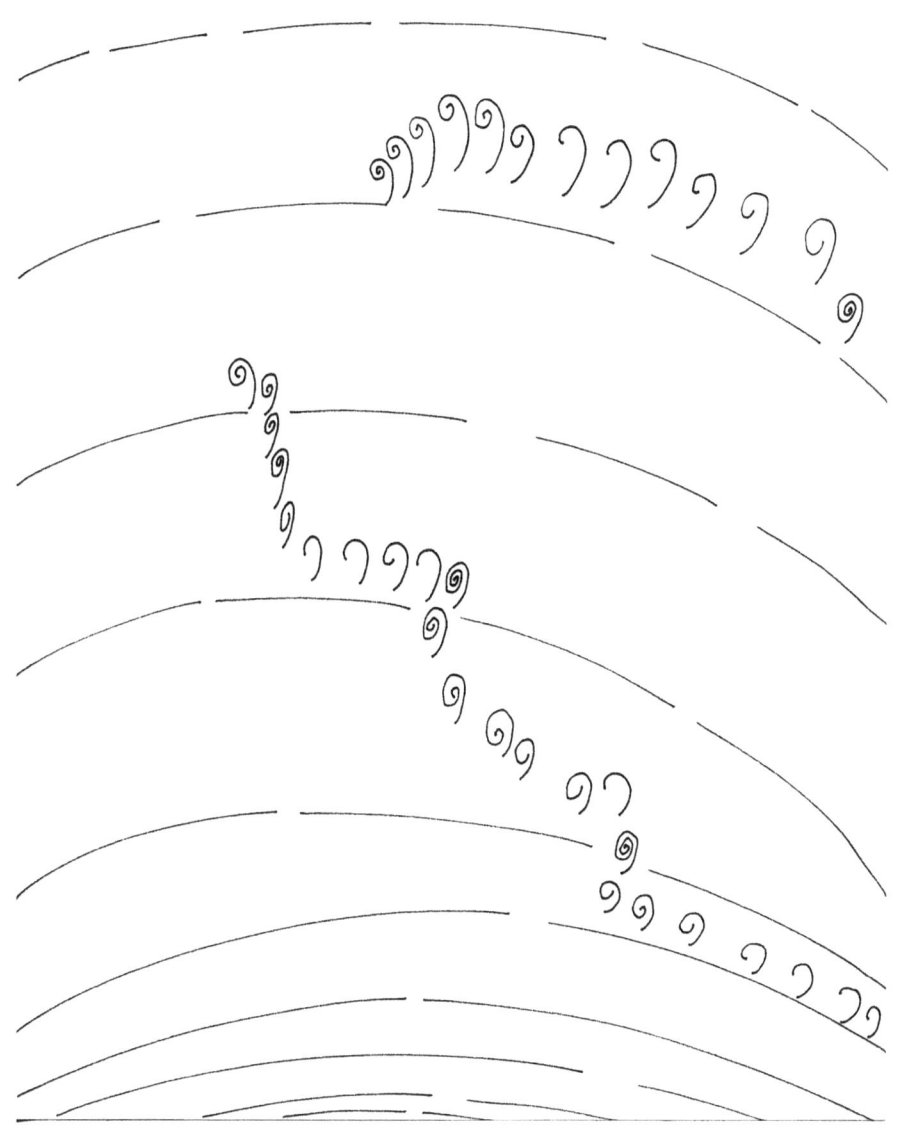

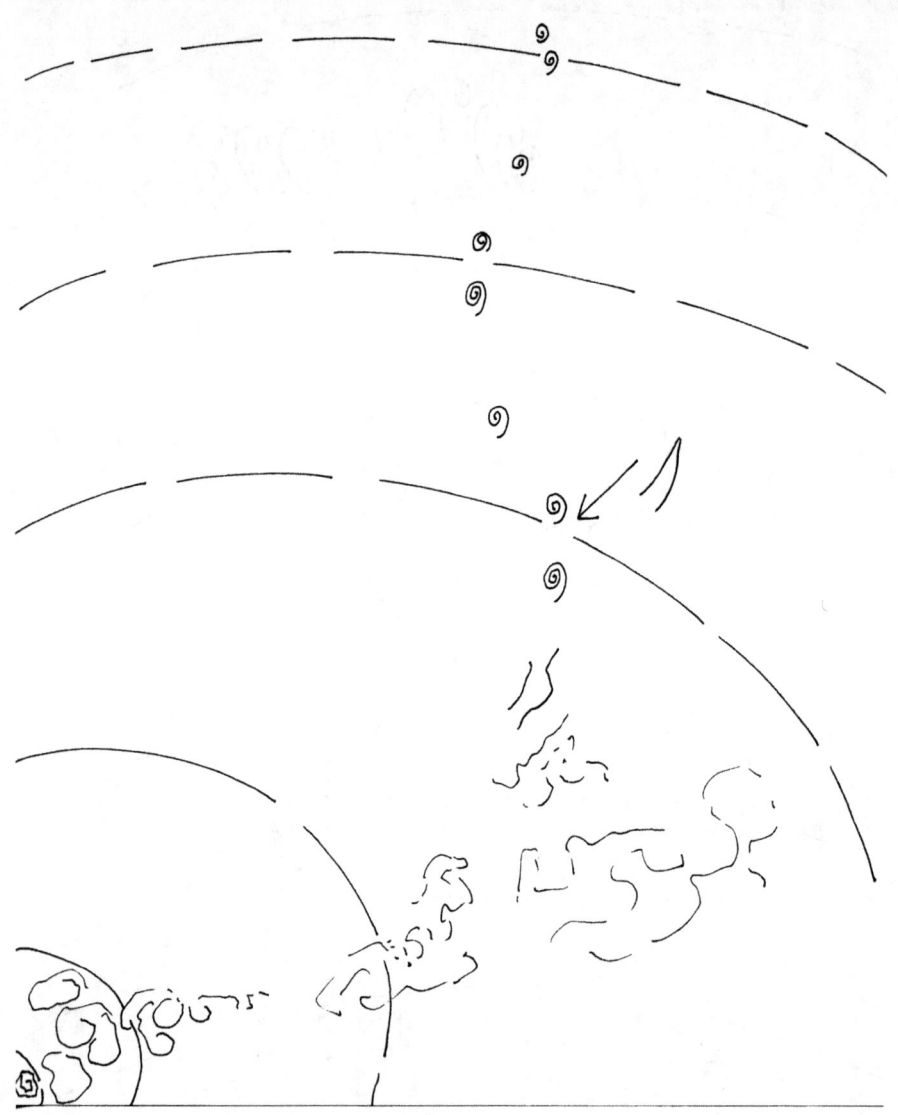

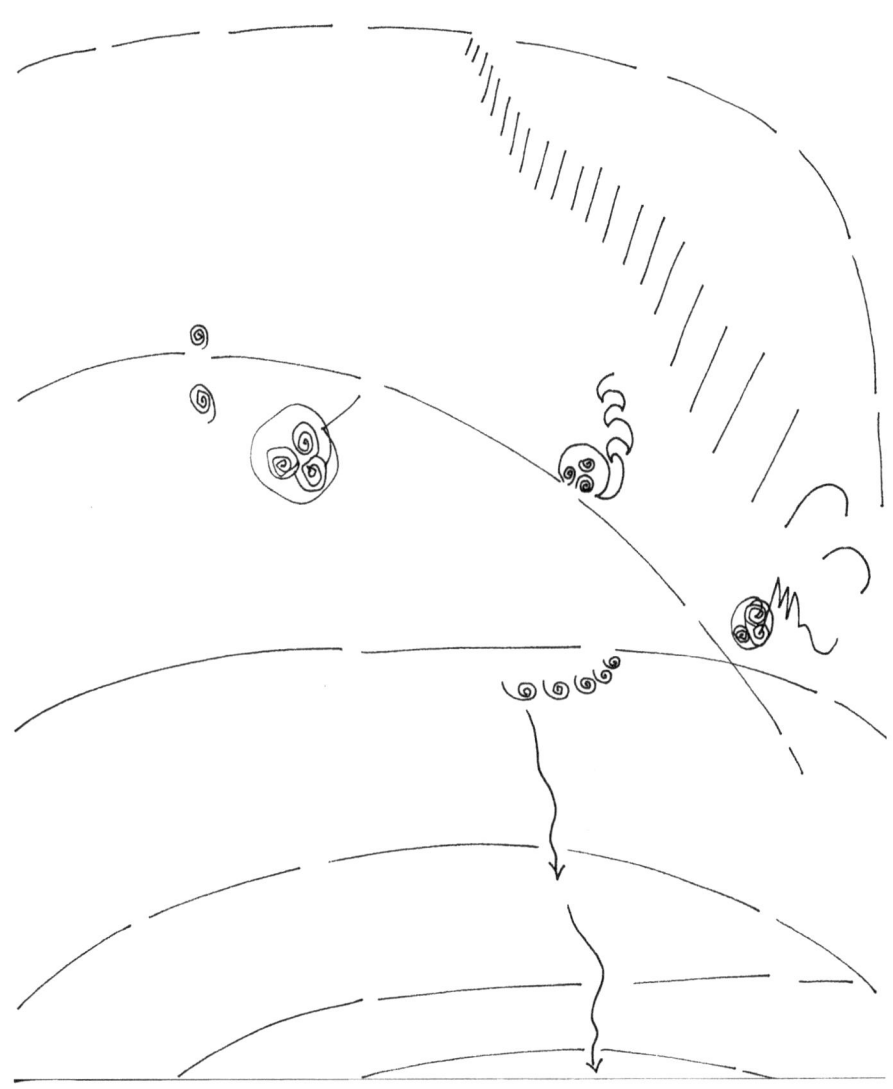

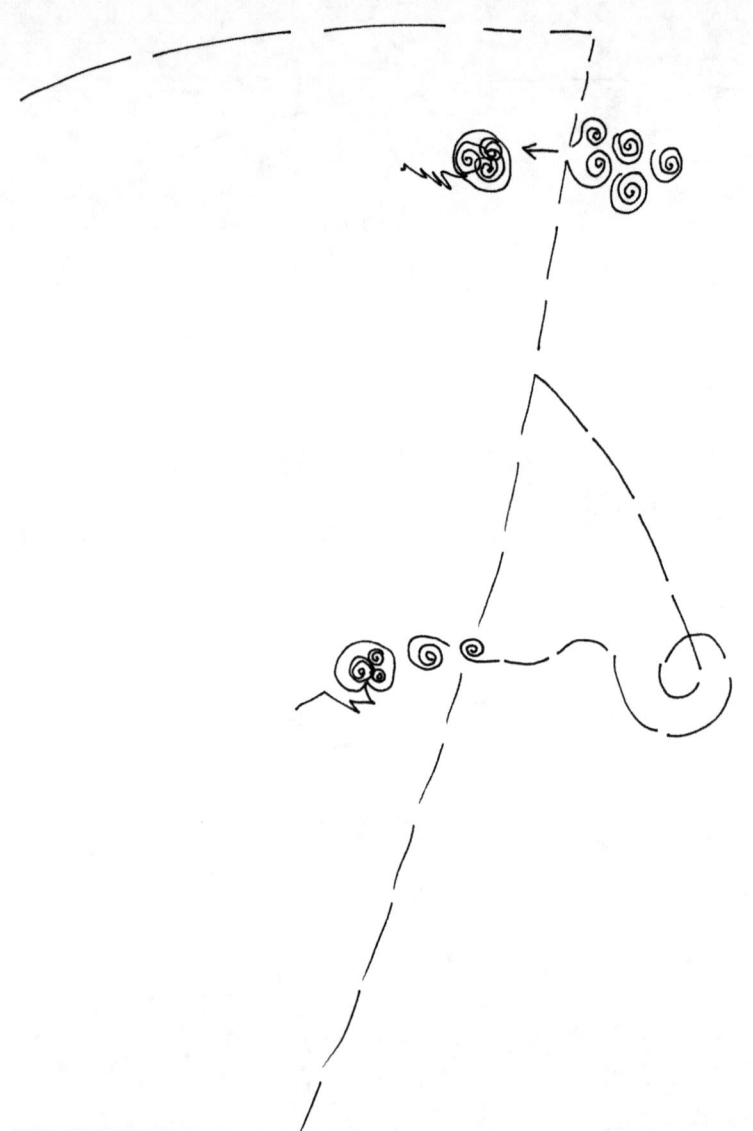

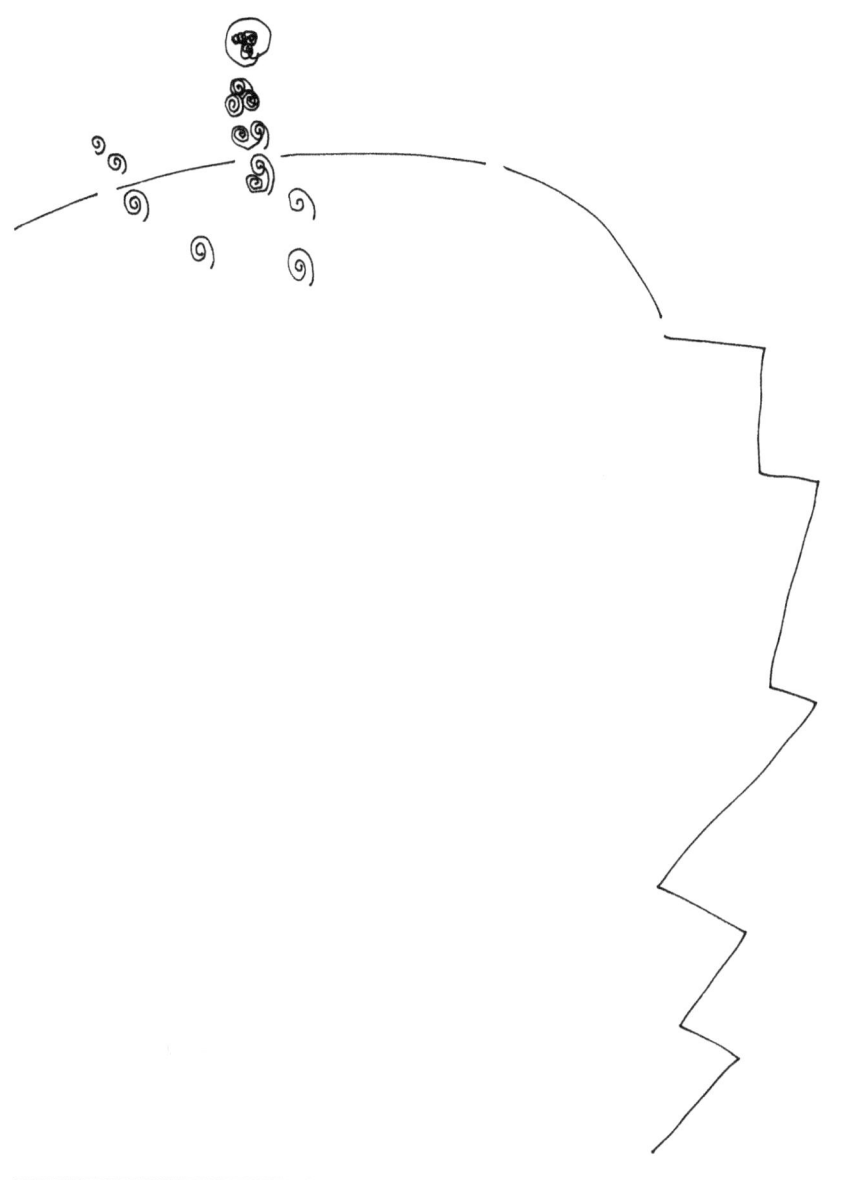

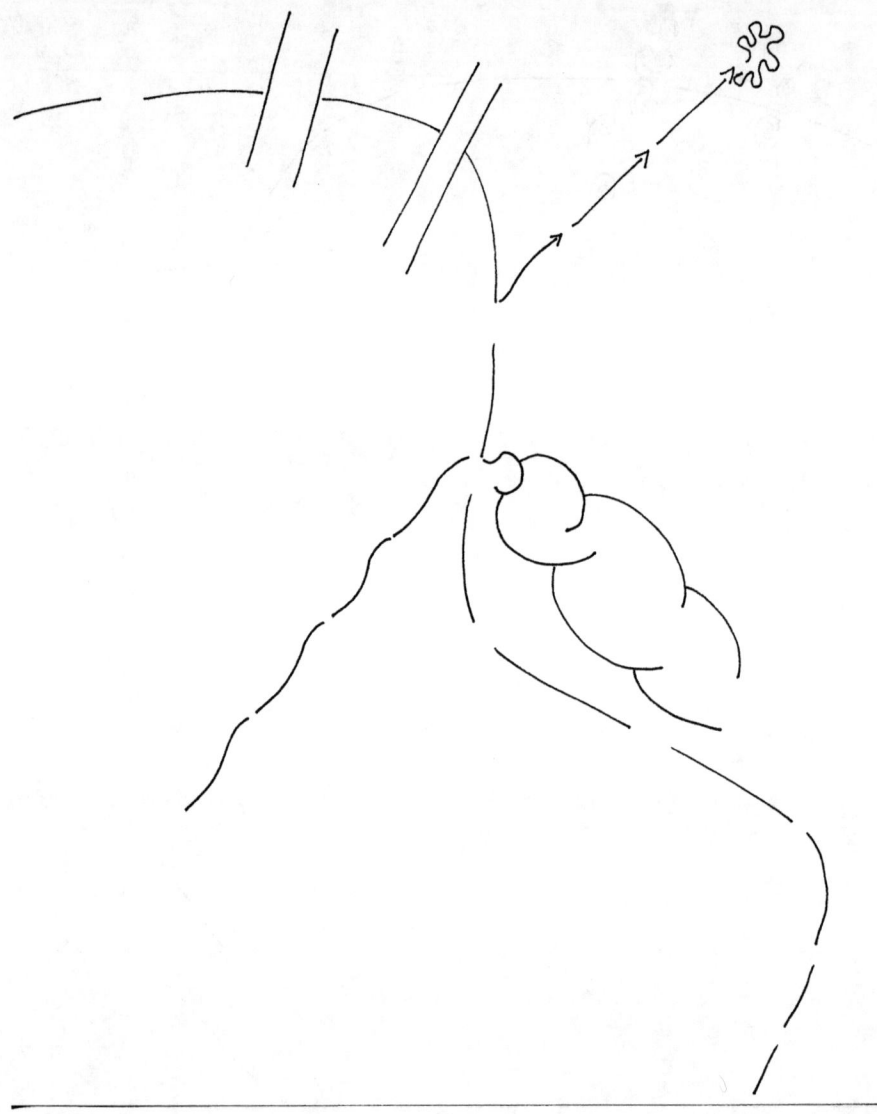

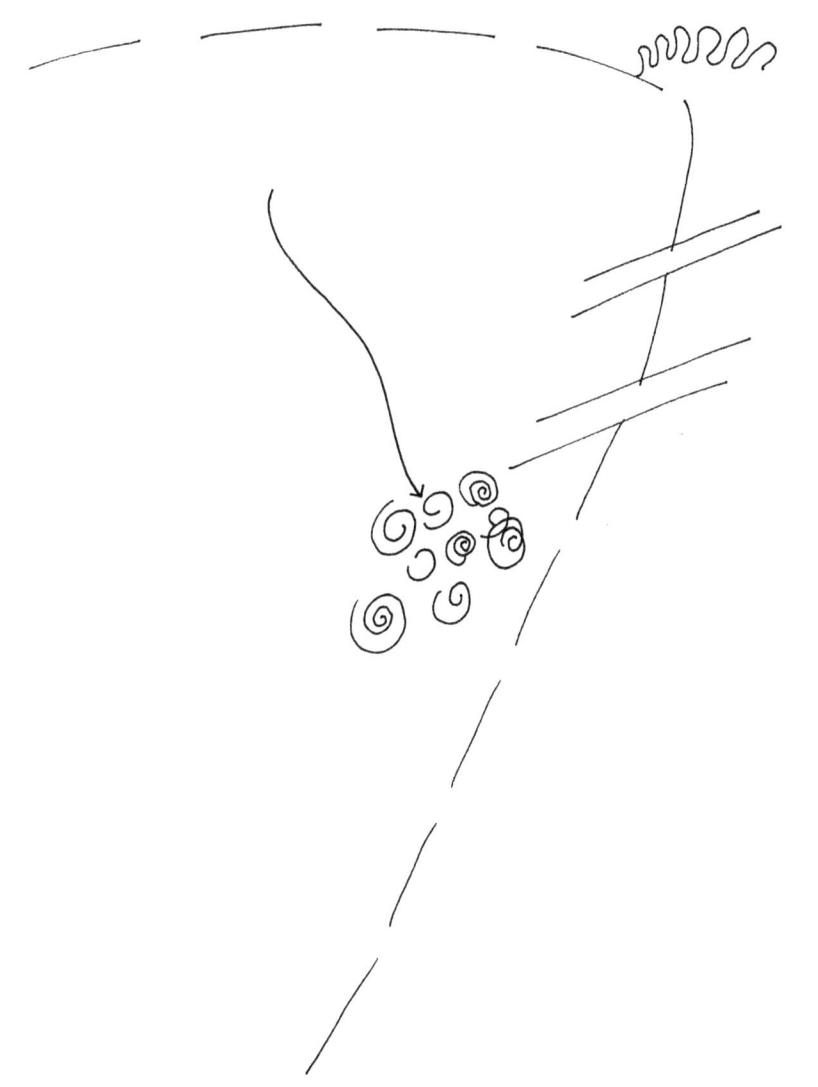

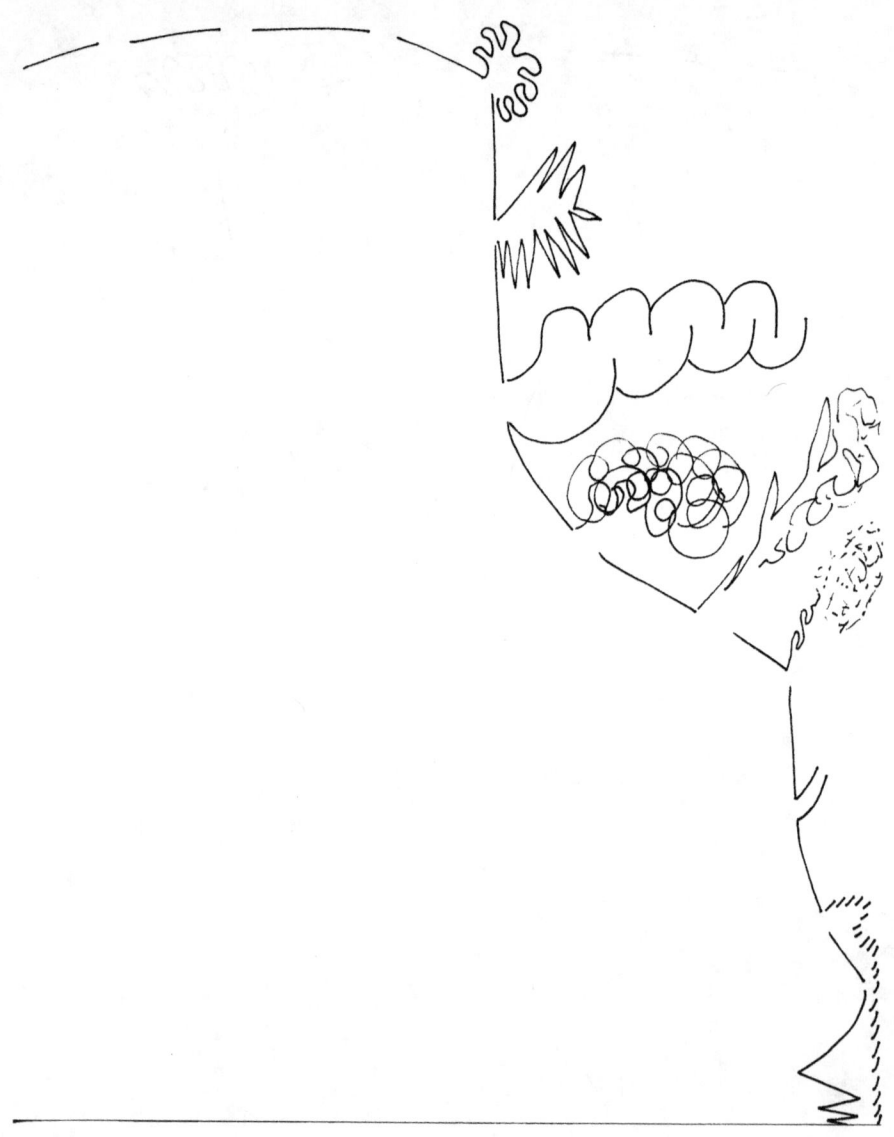

CONTINUED IN VOLUME 4

www.ingramcontent.com/pod-product-compliance
Lightning Source LLC
Chambersburg PA
CBHW080657190526
45169CB00006B/2150